Chronic
Fatigue
Unmasked 2000

About the Author

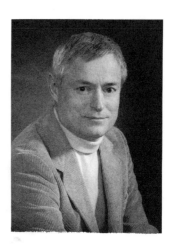

G.E. Poesnecker, D.C., N.D., has long been recognized as a leader in the alternative health movement. An innovative clinical diagnostician and therapist, he became the first Director of the internationally recognized Clymer Health Clinic in Quakertown, Pennsylvania in 1969, a position he held until 1983. He continues his pioneering work in Chronic Fatigue Syndrome at Clymer Healing Research Center in Quakertown.

Dr. Poesnecker has written several other books on healing and philosophy including, *It's Only Natural, Adrenal Syndrome, Creative Sex, A Guide for the New Renaissance, The Circle of Lives* and *In Search of Love and Wisdom, One Flesh, In Search of Health and Happiness* and *Nature Cure 2000*. He is the father of five children, several of whom have followed him into the health field; a skilled photographer, a typographer who typesets his own books and the Director General and minister of the Church of the Living Christ in Quakertown.

For over forty years Dr. Poesnecker has helped sick and tired patients overwhelmed by unremitting stress to overcome their symptoms and weaknesses with a comprehensive program aimed at supporting and regenerating the glandular and immune systems. This book describes in detail his successful program. For those who would like to contact Dr. Poesnecker, he can be reached at Clymer Healing Research Center, 5916 Clymer Road, Quakertown, PA 18951, telephone 1-800-300-5168.

Chronic Fatigue

Unmasked 2000

This Pioneering Classic has been completely
revised to encompass the latest successful
therapies and concepts of what Dr. Poesnecker
originally called "Today's most misunderstood,
mistreated and ignored health problem"

Gerald E. Poesnecker, N.D., D.C.
Foreword by Harold E. Buttram, M.D.

Humanitarian Publishing Company
Quakertown, PA 18951

Table of Contents

Foreword

Third Edition (1999)

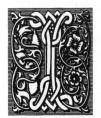N the last six years many changes have occurred in the nature of the of the public perception of Chronic Fatigue Syndrome (CFS). There has even been a certain degree of movement in the medical community itself, but most of this has been among a few physicians who have taken the time to really attempt to understand the nature of this condition and not, as the vast majority of their fellow practitioners do, attempt to squeeze CFS patients into a known condition that can be treated by tried and true drug therapy.

Whereas six years ago most CFS patients were still considered to be malingering or just downright lazy by most physicians, they are now looked upon as "depressed" and placed on a variety of antidepressants. The use of antidepressants in CFS is like the use of NSAIDs in arthritis. They treat the symptoms but do nothing to correct the real cause of the condition.

At least in the past doctors did little to interfere with the course of CFS, and the patient was free to seek a realistic cure, but now with the antidepressant therapy, the patient may be soothed in believing that he is being adequately treated and not seek physiological help before the condition has reached a very advanced stage. It is somewhat ironic to consider that this is an exact reflection of usual complaint of my colleagues that the alternative therapist is preventing the patient from receiving the correct treatment for various conditions as given by orthodox practitioners. Thank goodness that there are medical men like Drs. David S. Bell, Paul R. Cheny and Charles W. Lapp who do understand CFS and know that it is not just another form of depression.

At a recent seminar at which both Drs. Bell and Lapp lectured, it was obvious from the audience reaction that most of the physicians attending attempted to fit CFS into paradigms they already understood rather than were willing to gain an understanding of a new paradigm. One physician at this seminar, apparently a psychiatrist, attempted to assure the audience that all youths with CFS were in reality sexually abused as young children. Dr. Bell, who has made the most complete study of children and CFS to date, let him know in no uncertain terms that in his extensive fifteen-year study he found no child abuse in any of his young patients.

This reticence of the medical establishment to accept the true nature of CFS is understandable if we take into consideration a few salient factors:

1. Chronic Fatigue Syndrome defies the present state of medical laboratory testing. All the known tests can be run on CFS patients and most of them are normal. That is not to say that there are not tests (see the ASI test in the body of this book) that can not only diagnose CFS but also tell us the exact stage the CFS patient is in and the correct required treatment, but with rare exceptions, these definitive CFS tests are not known to the rank and file medical practitioner.

2. The proper care of CFS reverses the present trend toward hands-off treatment of the patient. CFS cannot be successfully treated at this time by "scientific" methods. CFS, more than any other common condition, requires that the physician practice the "Art" of medicine as well as the science. This is such a departure for the modern physician that it is almost impossible for him to shift gears to put himself into this mode of operation. This lack of the Art of medicine is one of the major reasons for the next factor, which is:

3. Frustration. At the end of the seminar mentioned above,

the doctors were asked to express their feelings regarding CFS. The nearly universal reply was one word—frustration. The reason for this is simple and understandable. CFS is all too often the result of modern medical treatment of individuals susceptible to the condition. The more these patients are given regular drug treatment, the worse they eventually become. It is not hard to see that frustration would develop in a doctor when everything he attempts to do to help his patient seems to make the patient worse. But that is the nature of CFS, and no doctor can really help a patient with this condition if he is not aware of this fact and does not adjust his treatment accordingly.

4. As alluded to in (3), there is much evidence to support the contention that some of the methods used by the orthodox medical profession have been among the major underlying causes of CFS in those susceptible to this condition. These methods include such things as the use of multiple vaccines in children, the overuse of antibiotics in all ages, the explosion of designer pharmaceuticals (that is, drugs based on chemical structures wholly alien to both our bodies and to Nature) and the mistreatment of CFS in the early readily treated stages.

I wish I could be as optimistic about the future of the medical community and CFS as was my counterpart in the 1993 Foreword of this book, but as a medical physician myself I know how hard it is to move the profession as a whole to a position that does not agree with its present practices. We all have heard of the treatment given Dr. Semmelweis when he attempted to have his collegues wash their hands between operations. They drove him insane before they finally accepted his rather obvious suggestion.

If it took so much time and effort to move the medical community to such a simple and nonthreatening change, we can only imagine how long it will take to entice them to give up some of their well-established and lucrative practices just to help prevent and cure CFS. We, who have followed this condition with a knowledge of Dr. Poesnecker's diagnostic and treatment methods, have seen it grow from a few isolated cases into a true epidemic. In the early years these patients were relatively easy to treat, but as the condition has progressed it has become more and more serious. Dr. Poesnecker's explanation of this is that the various man-made stresses on all mankind are continuing to increase day by day, and as they increase they are able to overwhelm the immune threshold of tolerance of more and more individuals, who then begin the CFS pattern. Those individuals who were already affected advance deeper into the condition and become increasingly difficult to return to normal.

While there are good efforts going on all over the world to treat CFS, I know of none that are as advanced as the efforts of Dr. Poesnecker. His methods are rather unusual when compared with the orthodox; but then, so is CFS. He has not only developed a successful treatment for CFS, but he has actually developed an entire new paradigm of medical protocol. It is unusual, but very effective. I am reminded of the comments the conductor George Szell made about the pianist Glen Gould when he first heard him sing along as he played Bach, "This man is a nut!" After he had listened a little longer, he added, "Ah, but this nut is also a genius."

Harold E. Buttram, M.D.
August 1998

Introduction

Third Edition

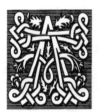S my interest in and treatment of Chronic Fatigue Syndrome (CFS) reaches its forty-second year it seems that my reputation among my fellow practitioners is changing from that of quack and charlatan to that of pioneer. Of course when I mention this fact to a patient I always add, "You know how you tell a pioneer, don't you? He's the one with all the arrows in his back."

In a more serious vein, this present edition of *Chronic Fatigue Unmasked 2000* is not just a reprint but a complete revision of the work. Many of the items and procedures discussed in the first two editions either are no longer available, or better methods have replaced them. During the interim between the second and this third edition we have kept our patients up-to-date by issuing monographs describing the latest tests and treatments that have become available for Chronic Fatigue Syndrome. The information in these monographs has been included in Appendix III of this new edition. You will also find here many new concepts about the condition as a whole. As the Chronic Fatigue Syndrome pandemic (yes, pandemic) spreads and intensifies, newer and more specific treatments are needed for its control, and we always do our best to keep on the cutting edge of all technologies related to this condition. Readers of this book who would like to keep up with our updates may do so in one of two ways: (1) Send us your name and address and we will put you on our list to send you new monographs as soon as they are issued or (2) contact our website, www.chronicfatigue.org, on a regular basis. All new monographs will be posted.

As I reread the Introduction to the 1993 edition of this work, I find that I still agree with the substance, but differ with some of the details. I don't know if it is practical to attempt to differentiate between Chronic Fatigue Syndrome and Chronic Fatigue Immune Dysfunction. The mere fact that a virus is the stress factor that triggers the Chronic Fatigue reaction does not seem to me now to be such an important distinction. The patient still needs to be treated the same as the regular Chronic Fatigue Syndrome patient. As the physician is able to build the immune system, the virus is taken care of naturally. I personally am very suspicious of drug viral therapy. As they are now finding in the treatment of AIDS, antiviral drugs tend to cause a mutation of the virus into a drug resistant form that might end up causing far more trouble than if they had not attempted to "kill" the virus in the first place. I realize that these views are somewhat heretical (so what else is new?), but more and more respectable researchers are coming to the same conclusions. Just remember, you heard it here first.

The two main bones of contention between myself and those medical doctors who are becoming more knowledgeable about Chronic Fatigue Syndrome have to do with the nature of the patient and the underlying cause of the disease. The others usually contend that (a) the patients are the same as everyone else except they have a strange new disease and (b) that the cause of this disease is some single factor (perhaps a yet-to-be-discovered virus such as HIV) and once this is discovered and overcome the disease will be a thing of the past. Like the belief in Santa Claus, I would love both concepts to be true, but my old-fashioned German-Norwegian hardheaded logic just won't let me do so.

Long experience with CFS has taught me that some persons are almost certain to develop this condition to some degree in their lives, while others will probably never fall victim to its ravages no matter what they do or how they live.

The immune system in the first group is weak and susceptible, while in the second it is inherently strong and vital. Therefore, I cannot agree with the contention that *anyone* can develop CFS. Long experience with this condition has proven to me that only a certain type of constitution is likely to develop this condition as we know it today. However, as CFS becomes more and more prevalent, I will qualify my previous conclusions to this degree: As the stresses of the world increase and as more and more individuals whose immune systems were compromised as children are placed (or place themselves) in positions of unremitting stress, the number of Chronic Fatigue Syndrome patients will increase greatly. This prediction is already being fulfilled with each passing day.

I believe the number of susceptible Chronic Fatigue Syndrome patients is increasing exponentially because their compromised childhood immune systems are reaching the end of their effective tether. When we are born into this world, we have certain very special immune units that can be used once and only once to fight off serious invaders. If these are wasted in adapting the immune system to the multiple disease organisms used in the rapid injection of manifold inoculations, the immune system will not have these units available in later life when they will be needed, and modern science has created an individual with a defective immune system who may become a prime candidate for later CFS.

As far as the virus theory of CFS is concerned, I feel the jury is still out. It really would be nice to find a quick, simple cure for this condition, but I still am not inclined to believe that such exists. A large percentage of my CFS patients have no history of such infections, but they do have a history of having pushed themselves beyond their strength time and time again until they could push no further. Therefore, I feel that even if such a virus were found, it would be helpful in only a small percentage of patients. My experience with CFS tells me that there are usually plenty of other reasons most patients develop this condition, and unless we reverse those reasons, that is, change the life-style that brought on the conditions in the first place, there is little hope of a real cure.

By the way, my good friend and mentor Dr. John Bastyr, mentioned in my 1993 Introduction, passed away a few years ago. He has not been forgotten, however. A college of Naturopathic healing has been established and named for him in Seattle, Washington.[1]

Gerald E. Poesnecker, N.D., D.C.
July 4, 1998

---

[1] John Bastyr College of Naturopathy.

Chapter One

The Nature of the Disease

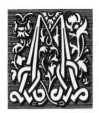Y more than forty years' experience has led me to believe Chronic Fatigue Syndrome (CFS) is a condition of the neurohormonal and immune mechanisms of the body that produces a weakening of the body's ability to respond to stress of all kinds. The most common symptoms produced by this condition are unexplained exhaustion sometimes alternating with spells of anxiety or panic, a tendency to be oversensitive and/or allergic to certain substances or environments, a lessening of the ability to reason rationally and to make decisions readily, a tendency toward low blood pressure, sensitivity to cold, poor circulation (cold hands and/or feet), and brain fag or other mental aberrations which can mimic a large variety of mental diseases. Individuals in the Countershock or Resistance stage of CFS (see Dr. Selye's chart in Chapter Five) may not suffer the fatigue, but will experience mostly the anxiety and/or panic symptoms until they enter the Exhaustion stage. Most patients with CFS have at least one of these symptoms, and some have all and many others besides.

This condition, to a lesser or greater degree, affects 20 to 25 percent of the American population. Fortunately, most of these are not severely afflicted, but today vast numbers of our people function at less than half their true potential because of CFS. Since it is the nature of the CFS patient to be a responsible, creative and productive citizen, the loss to America caused by this condition is significant.

As common as this condition is, only in the last few years has it been recognized, and it still is rarely treated effectively by most practitioners of the orthodox medical persuasion. In my early editions of this work, I called this condition, "The most ignored disease in the country today." Unfortunately, while the condition is not as ignored now as it once was, it does seem that the patients still are. A patient of mine, who is a vice president of a most prestigious university in Philadelphia, went to three of the best-known medical centers in Philadelphia with the symptoms of CFS. They all agreed that he had CFS, but they were equally unanimous in assuring him that they didn't know anything he, or they, could do to help his condition. Both he and his wife later came to us as patients and in a few weeks both were much improved.

Personally, I think that much of this medical apathy has been produced by the general vagueness of this disease's character, by the neurotic-like symptoms of its victims and by the slow and tortuous path of its correction even with the best and most advanced therapies. In our Clinic, I always meet the newly diagnosed CFS patient with mixed feelings. I am on one hand pleased to know that the patient has started on the road to becoming useful and productive again instead of languishing in a low-functioning state; on the other hand, I always groan a bit inside when I think of the amount of care, time and constant loving support that will be necessary to carry this patient through the seemingly unproductive early stages of treatment. With perseverance, however, all patients respond, and in the end they prove to be among our most appreciative patients. This thought—at times, this thought alone—gives us the ability and the strength to carry on with the CFS patient.

There seems to be a quirk in many doctors which, perhaps more than anything else, may explain their seemingly conspiratorial refusal to recognize CFS. Most physicians, in order to function as stable human beings, require a certain amount of personal ego satisfaction when they treat a patient. Even though there are vast fields of disease which are complete mysteries to modern medicine, the average day-to-day working physician often feels he must, at least in some manner, examine all the symptoms and problems that confront him. If he cannot rationally explain them, he must make up explanations, and if he cannot cure his patients, he must find some way to place the blame for his lack of understanding, knowledge and ability on the patient or on the circumstances. In the early days of medicine, physicians had ready explanations for causes of symptoms and ailments which were presented to them. The fact that today we realize that most of these early explanations were ridiculous has not prevented the medical profession from continuing this practice. To witch doctors, all diseases are caused by demons that inhabit their patients. Their job, of course, is to exorcise these demons. The "scientific" physician, when confronted with a patient who displays the symptoms of CFS, has a ready answer: "The patient is depressed, neurotic, mildly psychotic, unmotivated or just bored with life." With that self-satisfied stance that can be a "badge of our tribe," the patient is given a tranquilizer, antidepressant or both, and with the fatherly advice to stop worrying and to go to work he is sent home. It is just as impractical to tell a tubercular patient to go and play football as it is to tell a CFS patient to stop worrying.

Am I exaggerating? Am I a little too hard on my medical contemporaries? One has only to remember that a short time ago patients were literally bled to death in an effort to satisfy this medical ego—our first president being among those to be so helped into the next world.

There is, however, a specific cause that produces these wrecks of human society, and there are ways of returning these people to active, productive lives. This book defines this disease, lists the various symptoms produced by this condition, assesses the various stresses that trigger and aggravate this ailment and outlines a comprehensive plan of treatment to overcome this insidious disorder.

This last paragraph was written in 1983 and I see no reason to alter it for this new 1999 edition. That is still what this book does and we trust that it does it better today than ever before.

The Adrenal Gland

Before proceeding with our discussion of Chronic Fatigue Syndrome, its causes and its treatment, let us consider the nature of the adrenal gland—the gland that our research has determined is the major culprit (or victim) of CFS. The adrenal sits like a bishop's cap on the top of each kidney; each weighs about as much as a nickel coin. The adrenal gland is recognized as one of the body's most important endocrine or ductless glands, that is, glands that produce hormonal or hormone-like substances and discharge them directly into the bloodstream. Each of the endocrine glands is subject to a chain of command. The pituitary gland, so-called master gland of the body, sends out stimulatory or trophic hormones which regulate each of the target endocrine glands, such as the adrenals, the thyroid or the reproductive glands. The pituitary in turn is regulated or controlled by the hypothalamus, which produces specific releasing factors for each of the pituitary trophic hormones. (Later in our text you will read more about this Hypothalamic–Pituitary Axis and its effect on CFS.)

The adrenal glands are composed of two parts—the medulla (inner portion) and the cortex (outer surrounding portion). The medulla fits inside the cortex like a walnut inside its shell. The medulla and cortex produce many substances, the most important of which are epinephrine (formerly called adrenaline), which is produced by the medulla, and various sterols, such as cortisone and aldosterone, produced by the cortex.

When the body is called upon to respond to stress, the adrenal gland is its primary agent and target. Stress on the body stimulates (probably by way of the sympathetic nervous system) the adrenal medulla to increase epinephrine production. This hormone increases the secretion of adrenocorticotrophin (ACTH) by the pituitary gland, which in turn activates the adrenal cortex to greater production of corticoids such as cortisone.

Diseases of the Adrenal Gland

Of primary concern in the discussion of CFS is its differentiation from Addison's disease (organic adrenal insufficiency) and from adrenal insufficiency secondary to hypopituitarism. The term Chronic Fatigue Syndrome as we use it here refers to a state of depletion of the adrenal glands in the absence of atrophy or destruction. In other words, it is a state of functional depletion, or exhaustion. This is in contrast to Addison's disease, in which there is physical atrophy or destruction of the adrenal glands, or to hypopituitarism, in which there is some form or degree of destruction of the pituitary gland. Both Addison's disease and hypopituitarism are relatively rare, whereas CFS as herein described is nowadays becoming more and more common.

Diagnosis

Until recently the standard diagnosis of Chronic Fatigue Syndrome was a matter of exclusion; that is, such diagnosis was justified only after other causes of chronic fatigue, exhaustion, weakness and lassitude had been ruled out. Fortunately, the biological and biochemical changes that underlie this syndrome are now much better understood than in our early editions of this work. Definitive tests are now available in the form of the Adrenal Stress Index™ (ASI), a series of tests that chart the adrenal gland output throughout an entire day in comparison with the DHEA (the substance from which the hormones are produced) and immune system levels. With this test it is possible to determine not only if the patient has CFS or not, but also just what stage of the condition he is in and what is the best treatment for a complete recovery.

Unlike CFS, most patients with pathological adrenal function may be fully assessed by standard laboratory tests which include serum cortisol levels and urinary corticosteroids. In Addison's disease, even in advanced adrenal destruction or atrophy, the resting or basal levels of these tests may be within the lower levels of normal. For this reason, a diagnosis of

Addison's disease may depend on results of a pituitary stimulation test in which corticotropin (ACTH) is injected into the patient. In normal persons a significant rise in serum cortisols follows ACTH injection, but in Addison's disease there is minimal or no response. In cases in which pituitary insufficiency is suspected, the metyrapone stimulation test is utilized. These tests are described in detail in standard medical texts.

Standard medical texts state that clinical adrenal insufficiency (Addison's disease) usually does not occur unless at least 90 percent of the adrenal cortex has been destroyed by idiopathic atrophy, granulomatous destruction, or some other form of destructive process. By the same token, currently available tests, including the ACTH stimulation test, may not show abnormal results except in the case of advanced disease or depletion. On the basis of present information, it would appear that these tests lack the sensitivity to detect or diagnose lesser degrees of adrenocortical depletion, as in CFS. Therefore, the condition of CFS is largely undetected by these orthodox measures. The ASI is still at this time not well known except in the alternative medical community.

Causes of the Condition

What causes this system breakdown? Why are some people affected and others not? There are two common causes of this condition. They are often mixed in the sufferer to the point that it is difficult to say which actually caused the disorder in any specific case. The two causes are hereditary weakness and overwhelming, unremitting stress. After more than forty years of working with this condition, I feel that inherent hereditary weakness of the system is probably the most consistent cause of the difficulty. The glandular weakness seems to be passed down from one generation to another, the most common relationship being from mother to daughter, although any genetic combination is possible. Without adequate treatment, each succeeding generation often becomes weaker than the previous generation. Therefore, in most CFS cases, the sufferer has inherited a lessened ability to adapt to the stresses of life. To make this more readily understandable to the patient, I usually refer to this situation as the inheritance of a weakened or poorly vascularized adrenal gland. While this is not entirely scientifically correct, there being other factors in a deficient general adaptive system, this is easy for the patient to comprehend and is not that far from the truth.

Some persons' adaptive mechanisms are so weak that no matter how they govern their lives, they are destined to have a problem with this system. Such a problem usually begins shortly after puberty from the stresses of the glandular changes which occur at this time. These patients come to us and say, "I've been tired as long as I can remember, Doctor. I never have had the energy or the ability to do what other people do with ease." The majority of hereditary adrenal cases, however, have sufficient adrenal functioning to live a relatively stable, normal life until a truly overwhelming, unremitting stress presents itself—a stress that exhausts the adaptive mechanism and finally throws these patients into full-blown CFS. These persons show the interplay of the two basic causes of CFS: first, a hereditary weakness of the basic adrenal system itself, and, second, unremitting stresses that are able to inhibit the normal functioning of the mechanism.

The combination of these factors, however, varies tremendously in any specific individual. For instance, as previously mentioned, it is possible for an individual to be born with such a weakened adaptive system that almost any of the normal adaptive needs of life can throw that person deeply into CFS at some point in his life. Patients with this weakness are to be greatly pitied, for until they receive proper treatment, they are never able to experience the real pleasures and satisfactions of life.

A larger number of individuals have some weakness of the adrenal system, but can live fairly normally until the stresses in their lives pile up to such a degree that they, too, will begin to manifest the symptoms of CFS. The majority of our patients fall into this category. With wise and dedicated treatment they can be returned to normal functioning, but will need to live within their adrenal ability if they desire to keep from returning to the CFS state.

Next, there are individuals who are blessed with a fairly normal adrenal mechanism, but who are unfortunate enough in life, as Shakespeare put it, "To suffer the slings and arrows of outrageous fortune," and to have stresses and pressures so enormous and so unresolved that the normally functioning adrenal system with which they are blessed is no longer capable of sustaining their needs. It eventually weakens and plunges them into some variety of CFS. These individuals should be the easiest to return to productive life, but this is not always the case. The main problem is that since they were healthy for so long, it is difficult to get them to make the needed changes in their life-style that are essential for their recovery.

Last, there are the fortunate persons whose adrenal or general adaptive mechanism is so strong that almost nothing in life can affect it. They are capable of going through all possible stresses, and therefore, at least in the past, have not succumbed to CFS, no matter what occurs. We say "in the past" because as the stresses of life continue to increase, it is possible that even the strongest adrenal may give way to CFS in time.

Most of us fall somewhere in between the extremes of the last category of individuals who possess a strong general adaptive mechanism and the first-mentioned case of the unfortunate patients with serious hereditary inadequacy.

Almost all of us feel the effects of temporarily lowered adrenal functioning at some time in our lives, usually following a bacterial or viral infection or after some particularly grueling mental or emotional stress. At such a time, we often experience a short-term weakness and inability to do our regular tasks as efficiently and as accurately as we would like. This is the result of acute adrenal exhaustion. If we are wise, at this time we will rest and not attempt to force ourselves to do more than our weakened ability readily allows. If we obtain sufficient sleep, stay on a healthful diet and do not force ourselves to work until our strength returns, our adrenal system will shortly regenerate. Now, imagine yourself constantly in this state of weakness and exhaustion and you will know what the CFS patient feels every day. In Chapter III of this book, "The Nature of the Patient," this state is discussed at great length.

As can be seen from the above discussion, CFS is due to a malfunctioning of the neurohormonal system of the body. It is caused by a breakdown of a physical component of the human system. Unfortunately, the vagueness of most of the symptoms produced by CFS leads the patient to feel that the main difficulty is one of a mental or emotional nature. Indeed, the symptoms of CFS are almost identical to those caused by anxiety, depression or various other mental conditions. When we are fearful or in a state of depression, these emotional states cause various glandular mechanisms of the general adaptive system to produce secretions which cause symptoms similar to mental disorders. Cold sweating, dry throat, rapid and irregular heartbeat, dizziness, cloudiness of the mind, nausea, flushing of various parts of the body, and so on can all be caused by various emotional effects on the general adaptive system. These symptoms are the body's attempt to prepare us for a possible threat which does not exist except in our fears. For instance, if we were out in the woods hunting, the cry of a wildcat behind us would create a certain sense of fear. This fear would cause the body to prepare for what is known as the "fight or flight" mechanism—either to fight this danger or to run away from it as rapidly as possible. When in our modern life we develop an emotional fear or apprehension, the body mechanism is not capable of distinguishing it from a true danger; therefore, through the glandular system, it prepares us in the same manner as if we needed to face a real danger. Since there is no real danger and subsequent action, we do not readily utilize the hormones which were pumped into our systems, and thus a variety of symptoms are produced as these hormones first register, intensify and then slowly dissipate.

Many modern psychologists and psychiatrists recommend physical activity such as running or jogging to help allay the symptoms of anxiety and similar difficulties. What is occurring, of course, is that the various anxiety-produced substances are being utilized by the physical activity and are not left lying around, as it were, to create more physical symptoms to aggravate the original anxieties further. This therapy has some merit, although it is not an answer to the original anxiety. In CFS, this same admixture which is produced by the anxious patient is produced by the weakened glandular system itself in an effort to bring its body hormone levels up to the normal level. Thus we have a situation in which a person is not necessarily anxious or emotionally distraught, and yet the physical weakness (CFS) produces symptom patterns which are almost identical to those produced in the nervous, neurotic individual.

Just imagine what can happen to the patient suffering from this condition who goes to the average physician! Since there are no specific laboratory tests that identify CFS in its earlier stages, the doctor finds no known disease process; and since the patient's symptoms mimic those of an emotional or mental difficulty, it is little wonder that the physician usually diagnoses the condition as mental anxiety. The patient is advised to stop worrying, told to go home and relax, given either a tranquilizer or an antidepressant or both, and summarily dismissed. This is not meant as criticism of the doctor, who followed recommended medical therapy; in fact, almost any competent medical authority not conscious of or skilled in the diagnosis and treatment of CFS would come to the same conclusion.

In our early years, by the time we saw most CFS patients they were convinced that they really were mental cases. They have been assured by their physicians, their friends and even their loved ones that there was nothing wrong with them that a change of mind, a change of the way that they look at their lives or a few tranquilizers would not help. This was not true then, nor is it true today. CFS patients are individuals with a true physical disorder as specific as if they had pneumonia or tuberculosis. You might as well tell the tubercular individual to stop coughing as to tell the CFS patient to stop worrying or to stop feeling so tired and do an honest day's work like any normal human being. Persons afflicted with CFS simply are not normal human beings; they are individuals with a real problem who need real treatment and real understanding.

An Ominous Triad

Thus CFS may be viewed as a triad, all three parts of which must be considered in every case: **First,** the heredity factor on which all prognosis or outcome is based. **Second,** the stress component which is composed of stresses that may cause the CFS or be caused by it. **Third,** the group of symptoms which due to the nature of the condition are not only caused by the condition, but can become stresses which further aggravate the condition.

> *Therefore, we can amplify our original definition by stating that CFS is that condition of the neurohormonal system which can be produced in an hereditarily weakened structure by a multitude of possible stresses which, in turn, cause a variety of symptom patterns which can in themselves eventually become stresses, thus creating a self-perpetuating disease—one that is able to feed upon its own symptoms.*

The whole condition sounds ominous and almost hopeless of resolution, and so it must seem to the afflicted patient. For it is a condition that not only can be triggered in sensitive people by ordinary stresses of life, but which actually produces its own stresses via its symptomatology. We might say it is a beast that flourishes on its own excrement. As we come to understand more about the character of this disease, we see why it is so neglected and also so prevalent.

To understand it more fully and to become knowledgeable in its treatment, we must comprehend the interplay and ramifications of its three sides: heredity, stresses, and symptoms.

Heredity

Little can be done about the inherited factor except to attempt to determine its extent, since all treatment and prognosis (length of treatment and chance of complete recovery) depend on this fact. If inherited weakness is great, treatment must be extensive and great efforts must be made to reduce all patient stresses to a minimum. Conversely, if the heredity factor seems slight, treatment and stress reduction can be much less stringent and a quick recovery can be assured.

There is unfortunately no simple, exact way to determine the degree of hereditary weakness in any specific case. However, a clinician with much experience can usually make a fair estimate from the case history. Three matters are of prime importance: the age at which the symptoms began, the severity of the symptoms and the amount of stress that was required to produce the symptoms. If the symptoms began early, were severe and seemed to set in with little or no appreciable external stress, the heredity factor is strong, and such a case will require the best and most extensive therapy we have.

As a general guide, we can say that the degree of inherited neurohormonal weakness is in direct proportion to the severity of the patient's symptoms and inversely proportional to the stresses involved and the age at which they began.

Stress

Much has been written here concerning stress, but little has been written to define stress. To understand the stresses that affect CFS—not only those that cause it but also those that exacerbate it—is to understand the syndrome itself.

A stress in this context can be defined as any factor that stimulates the general adaptive system. These stresses may be divided into several types:

First, those stresses that would affect all human beings somewhat alike, *i.e.*, cold, heat, physical exertion, infectious diseases, toxic substances, malnutrition and such things as exposure to war, flood, earthquake and fire.

Second, stresses that are individual due to personal background and experience. For instance, you may have a relative to whom you owe a large sum of money that you are unable to repay. Word of his return from a long journey may gladden the hearts of the rest of his family, but it can strike fear and consternation in yours because of the debt. This example of personal duress is the type of unseen stress that is usually the most difficult to diagnose and correct.

Third, stresses that develop from the condition itself. The CFS usually causes a weakened digestive function, which in turn has an effect on the pancreas to produce a hypoglycemic condition which in turn produces more stress. This weakened digestion also allows many foods to enter the bloodstream incompletely broken down, thereby stimulating the body to produce antibodies to attempt neutralization of the foreign substance (leaky gut syndrome). These antibodies, when they next contact this food substance, produce certain end products that may act as cerebral allergens, causing a variety of stress symptoms. These are only two of the stresses caused by this condition of the adaptive mechanism, but the list is long and readily shows the self-perpetuating nature of CFS.

A full understanding of the stresses involved in CFS is vital to recovery because all treatment is based on two simple principles on which the physician and the patient must work together. One, do everything possible to build strength into the adaptive mechanism, and two, remove as many stresses from this mechanism as possible. Unless the nature of the stresses are understood, they cannot be removed from a person's life. Some stress admittedly is useful, but long experience has taught me that no matter how hard a physician and a patient work, there will always be some stresses left. It was Benjamin Franklin who said, "Those who have nothing to worry about will worry about nothing."

Symptomatology

Symptoms of CFS are unique—not so much because of their basic character, for these are symptoms common to other conditions, but because they themselves can have a profound effect on the course and progress of the disease. To understand this facet of CFS, let us examine a typical patient. Let's take a working mother who is developing the condition and who of late has been experiencing unusual and unexplainable symptoms, such as strange tinglings, dizziness, mild nausea, the inability to concentrate, difficulty in remembering and in making decisions, being constantly and usually tired, digestive disturbances, apprehensions and anxieties that do not seem to have a basis in fact but that come sweeping over her for no apparent reason. Every little thing seems like a mountain to her, every cry of one of her children sounds like a screaming siren in her ear, every request of her husband seems like an unwarranted demand. Why would she not be anxious? Why would she not wonder if she is losing her sanity? Why would she not manifest all forms of worries and fears which by their very nature create further stresses that in turn worsen the CFS, which creates more symptoms, and so on, ad infinitum?

As we have described, the symptoms of CFS produce a snowballing effect, and unless this effect is controlled, there is little hope of helping the patient. Once the worse CFS symptoms begin, they are often sufficient in themselves to perpetuate the condition regardless of outside stresses.

In order to truly treat this condition successfully, all the above factors must be taken into consideration. An entire new paradigm of doctor–patient relationship needs to be established. No doctor can do more than about half the work needed to overcome this condition—the rest is up to the patient. He must come to understand the condition and work in harmony with his physician. The doctor needs to take the reins of the case but must hold them loosely so that the patient can learn to overcome that which is in his province.

Chapter Two

History of the Disease

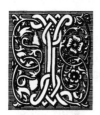N the past as in the present there have been physicians who were not afraid to investigate the true nature of the functional adrenal weakness that modern medicine calls Chronic Fatigue Syndrome (CFS). The first truly clear-thinking researcher in this field was Charles E. de M. Sajous, M.D., LL.D., Sc.D. A Fellow of the American College of Physicians and of the American Philosophical Society, professor of therapeutics at Temple University in Philadelphia, professor at the Medico-Chirurgical College, and clinical lecturer at Jefferson Medical College, he produced a text in 1903 entitled *The Internal Secretions and the Practice of Medicine.*[1]

In his book, he credited the physician Brown-Sequard as first bringing attention to the importance of the adrenal glands, in 1856. It was, however, through the experimental research work of Dr. Sajous himself, in our own city of Philadelphia, that the full significance of the adrenal mechanism, and particularly that part concerning the modern CFS, was brought into full realization. In his book he devoted an entire chapter to functional hypoadrenia, much of which I include here, not with the assumption that all of its conclusions are accurate nearly ninety years later, but to show the

---

[1]Sajous, Charles E. de M. *The Internal Secretions and the Practice of Medicine.* Philadelphia, F. A. Davis Company, 1903. (10th ed., 1922)

amount of knowledge accepted as standard medical information and procedure at that time.

According to Dr. Sajous:

"The adrenals playing so important a role in the maintenance of the life process itself, it is obvious that, apart from any organic lesion in these organs, any marked depression of their functional activity should manifest itself by symptoms corresponding with this depression. To the symptom-complex of this condition I have given the name of 'functional hypoadrenia' [what I later called "the Adrenal Syndrome"] to distinguish it from the forms due to destructive disorders of the adrenals, which constitute Addison's Disease and offer, of course, a far graver prognosis. As a definition of this condition, I would submit that 'functional hypoadrenia' is the symptom-complex of deficient activity of the adrenals due to inadequate development, exhaustion by fatigue, senile degeneration, or any other factor which, without provoking organic lesions in the organs or their nerve paths, is capable of reducing their secretory activity. Asthenia, sensitiveness to cold and cold extremities, hypotension, weak cardiac action and pulse, anorexia, anemia, slow metabolism, constipation, and psychasthenia are the main symptoms of this condition. [Certainly sounds like CFS, doesn't it?]

"The field covered by 'functional hypoadrenia' is necessarily a vast one, since it includes the asthenias so often met within the four main stages of life: infancy, childhood, adulthood, and old age, usually attributed to a 'weakness' or 'exhaustion,' and often 'neurasthenia,' which have been traced to no tangible cause. All I can submit herein, therefore, is a cursory analysis of the subject." [We feel that so-called neurasthenia was what CFS was known as in the early days of this century.]

Hypoadrenia in Infancy and Childhood

In discussing functional hypoadrenia of infancy and childhood, Dr. Sajous pointed out that, although the adrenals at birth are one-third the size of the kidney, and therefore relatively large, their functions are limited to the carrying on of the vital process, at least during the first year of life. During this time the mother's milk supplies the antitoxic products capable of protecting the infant against the destructive action of poisons. Dr. Sajous stressed the protective influence of mother's milk:

"It is an important function of the mother to transfer to the suckling, through her milk, immunizing bodies, and the infant's stomach has the capacity, which is afterwards lost, of absorbing these substances in active state. The relative richness of the suckling's blood in protective antibodies as contrasted with the artificially fed infant explains the greater freedom of the former from infectious disease."

He cited as striking proof of this immunizing function J.E. Winters' statement regarding the siege of Paris in 1870-1871 during the Franco-Prussian War: "While the general mortality was doubled, that of infants was lowered 40 percent, owing to mothers being driven to suckle their infants."

Children have a predilection to certain infectious diseases not only during infancy, but through at least their first ten years. Dr. Sajous stated that mother's milk helps provide protection to the suckling against such diseases; vulnerability in older children is overcome as the adrenals, with other organs, acquire the power to supplant the mother in contributing antitoxic bodies to the blood. These facts, Dr. Sajous stressed, point to the adrenals and other prominent organs, whose inadequate development explain the special vulnerability of children to certain infections. He believed that degrees of this hypoadrenia cause a child to be more or less liable to infection. He continued:

"That degrees of hypoadrenia exist in children is in reality a familiar fact to every physician when the signs of this condition are placed before him. The ruddy, warm, hard-muscled, heavy, out-of-door, romping child with keen appetite and normal functions is one in whom the adrenals are as active as the development commensurate with its age will permit. He is ruddy and warm because oxidation and metabolism are perfect and the blood pressure sufficiently high to keep the peripheral tissues well filled with blood; his muscular, skeletal, cardiac, and vascular systems are strong because, in addition to being well-nourished, they are exercised and well-supplied with the adrenal secretion, which ... sustains muscular tone. As normal outcome of this state, we have constant stimulation of the functional activity of the adrenals. The muscular exercise and maximum food intake involve a demand for increased metabolism and oxidation, and the resulting greater output of wastes imposes upon the adrenals, as participants in the oxidation and auto-protective processes, greater work, more active growth and development, with increase of defensive efficiency as normal result.

"The pale, emaciated, or pasty child with cold hands and feet, flabby muscles, whose appetite is capricious or deficient—the pampered house plant so often met among the rich—represents the converse of the healthful child described, just as does the ill-fed, perhaps overworked child of the slums. The emaciation, the cold extremities, indicate deficient oxidation, metabolism, and nutrition owing to the torpor of the adrenal functions; the pallor is mainly due to a deficiency of the adrenal principle in the blood and to the resulting low blood pressure, which entails retrocession of the blood from the surface. This child is not ill, but the hypoadrenia which prevails normally, owing to the undeveloped state of its adrenals, is abnormally low and it is vulnerable to infection."

Sajous believed that all conditions which in the adult tend to produce functional hypoadrenia affect the child at least to the same extent.

Hypoadrenia in the Adult

"Adults in whom adrenals may be inherently weak do not, as in hypothyroidia, show signs of myxedema; but their circulation and heart action are feeble, they tend to adiposis and show other signs of hypoadrenia. I have witnessed suggestive bronze spots in such cases. As a rule, however, the development of the adrenals in adults is an accomplished fact—as also that of their co-workers in the immunizing process, the thyroid and pituitary.... The adrenals, fully capable of sustaining oxidation and metabolism up to highest standard in all organs, also preserve the efficiency of all other defensive resources, including phagocytosis, with which the body is endowed to their highest level. On the whole, the normal adult whose adrenals function normally is relatively resistant to infection. The infrequency with which the physician is infected, notwithstanding daily exposure in his professional work, attests to this fact."

Dr. Sajous explained that functional hypoadrenia appears when irrespective of any disease, as the result of the vicissitudes of life, the adrenals are exhausted by excessive secretory activity that exaggerated labor or exercise—fatigue—imposes upon them. He cited a striking difference between patients with Addison's disease and those with other types of illness whose muscles are organically normal: signs of fatigue appear quickly and muscular impotence asserts itself in functional hypoadrenia patients, but, for example, in an advanced case of tuberculosis the patient may be able to show appreciable muscular strength. He used other illustrations of the influence of adrenal secretion over muscular tone to show the close relationship between fatigue and the functions of the adrenals:

"The unusual prevalence of disease among soldiers in the field is, of course, partly due to the defective sanitation that a campaign entails; but fatigue—particularly that due to heavy marching, carrying heavy accoutrements—is, in my opinion, an important predisposing cause, through its influence upon the adrenals. Not only are these organs called upon to sustain general oxidation and metabolism at a rate exceeding by far that which amply suffices for normal avocations, but the fact that ... they also serve to destroy the toxic products of muscular activity constitutes another cause of drain upon their secretory resources."

From studies of other investigators into the influence of fatigue on adrenal function in animals he noted that debility from any source—starvation, loss of blood, or other factors—makes the body vulnerable to disease. In a healthy animal, an injection of combined toxin and antitoxin resulted in no harm, but in an animal weakened by starvation or slight bleeding, death usually followed such an injection, with all the signs of poisoning by the toxin, including congested adrenals.

He pointed out the relationship between the adrenal gland and infection, adding that hypoadrenia from any source weakens the body so that it becomes vulnerable to disease. Among humans, he pointed to deficient food and excessive work as causes of the disease. Other important morbid factors in this condition, according to Sajous, include masturbation and excessive venery. He wrote:

"The pallor and asthenia witnessed in these cases, so far unexplained, can readily be accounted for if, as I believe, the liquid portion of the semen is rich in adrenal principle. This is suggested by the fact that spermin, the purest of testicular preparations, given the same tests, acts precisely as does the adrenal principle. The latter is an oxidizing body acting catalytically; it resists all temperatures up to, and even, boiling; it is insoluble in ether and practically insoluble in absolute alcohol, and gives the guaiac, Florence, and other heamin tests. Now spermin not only raises the blood pressure, slows the heart and produces all other physiological effects peculiar to the adrenal principles, but its solubilities are the same; it gives the same tests; it resists boiling. Moreover, it is regarded in Europe as a powerful 'oxidizing tonic' and has been found equally useful in disorders in which adrenal preparations had given good results. The inference that spermin consists mainly of the adrenal product suggests that it is not specific to the testes, but instead, a constituent of the blood at large; not only did this prove to be the case, but it was found in the blood of females as well as in that of males."

Hypoadrenia in the Aged

To Dr. Sajous, the ductless glands greatly influence old age. He wrote:

"All living organic matter is subjected, after more or less precarious periods of growth and adult existence, to one of decline and final disintegration. This applies particularly to the adrenals, if their functions are, as I hold, to sustain oxidation and metabolism, the fundamental process of the living state. Indeed, the senile state may be said to be as evident in these organs as it is in the features of the aged."

He quoted from investigators who had found that fat occurred in increasing quantities in the adrenal fibrous tissue between the cortex and medulla in very old animals and in the medulla of aged individuals. A marked—occasionally very great—reduction was found in the size of adrenals in the aged. In a study in which adrenals of three young men were compared with those of aged individuals, the adrenals in the young were well developed and in "full bloom," while in the aged they were shrunken and deficient, showing lowered activity, implying a lessening of the vital process the adrenal glands sustain.

"The asthenia of old age," he continued, "thus finds a normal explanation in the defective supply of adrenal secretion-precisely as it does in Addison's Disease. In fact...atrophy of the glands in the young may produce this disease." To Dr. Sajous, old age was caused by degeneration of the ductless glands. He believed that a condition of autointoxication existed in old age "quite in keeping with a decline in the antitoxic power shown by the adrenals." He also found a functional relationship between the adrenals and the thyroid in the genesis of old age.

Regarding the causation of old age, Sajous quoted an earlier researcher, Lorand: "It is evident...that all hygienic errors of diet or any kind of excess will bring about their own punishment, and that premature old age, or a shortened life, will be the result. In fact, it is mainly our fault if we become senile at 60 or 70, and die before 90 or 100."

As Seneca said, "Man does not die, he kills himself."

Summary of Sajous' Work

Sajous, then, believed that the lesions to which the adrenals are subjected during infections and autointoxication from birth to the last day of life greatly shorten life by limiting the functional area of the organs through the local fibrosis they entail. "It is quite probable," he wrote, "that centenarians owe their prolonged longevity mainly to integrity of their adrenals." To this end he saw hygiene, particularly its influence on the prevention of infectious disease, "as one of the most useful of sciences" because it helps prevent even seemingly benign diseases (diseases from which people recover), which "in the end shorten our existence by compromising the integrity of the organs which sustain the vital process itself."

Sajous discussed also the prophylaxis and treatment of the hypoadrenal condition. While much of the prophylaxis he discussed is not germane to the present day, he made several pertinent comments. In discussing prevention of hypoadrenia in infants, for example, he said:

"In infants, we should by every possible means prevent infection or intoxication to preserve the integrity of their adrenals and other auto-protective organs. The key of the whole situation lies in the fact that...nearly all the cases and nearly all the deaths are in bottle-fed babies. Physicians are, as a rule, entirely too ready to yield to the demands of social and other claims put forth by mothers who do not wish to nurse their offsprings. The responsibility assumed by both mother and physician under these circumstances is overlooked. I cannot but hope that if this continues, and the sacrifice of countless infants proceeds, laws may be enacted to prevent it by imposing upon the physician the duty of submitting to the State authorities a certificate in which sound reasons shall alone account for his consent to a departure from Nature's methods which entails deaths untold...The death rate among foundlings in New York City reached almost 100 percent until wet nurses were provided.... Many...authorities have written forcibly upon this subject, but seemingly to no avail. The holocaust continues."

Dr. Sajous devoted several pages to proving that mother's milk contains antitoxic substances that are not present in the bottled variety. Surprisingly, only in the last few years has so-called modern medical science caught up with Dr. Sajous.

In referring to the prophylaxis and treatment of the adult patient, Sajous discussed the importance of rest and of what physical stress with inadequate rest can do to the weakened adrenal gland. This factor has changed little to this day. He goes on to state:

"The influence of excessive fatigue on the adrenals, we have seen, is such as to weaken greatly their functional activity and, therefore, their oxygenizing and immunizing functions of the blood. The main harmful feature in this connection is the relative deficiency of rest, which means, from my viewpoint, inadequate opportunity afforded the adrenals to recuperate. This, of course, should be proportionate to the amount of strain imposed upon these organs, and the resistance of which they are capable. It is probably owing to lack of this that apparently strong men are often the first to "give out" in forced marches. The physical examination being based mainly upon the *status praesens*, and the adrenals being necessarily (for we are now dealing with a new line of thought) [Apparently still new today! - Author] overlooked as factors, there is marked inequality in the resistance of the men to strain. This applies as well to the pathogenesis of chronic disorders. In a personal analysis of 40 cases of hay fever, for instance, the severity of the disease corresponded to a considerable degree with the number of children's diseases the patient had had, the worst cases having had six of these diseases in comparatively quick succession." [Even here the child was not subjected to more than one disease at a time as is done at present in the use of multiple vaccines.]

To Dr. Sajous, this suggested the need of ascertaining the number and severity of children's and other diseases to which a recruit in the armed forces had been subjected and to add this factor to others in deciding upon his admission to the service or the arm to which he is to be assigned. He continued:

"The mounted man suffers less from actual fatigue than the infantry man who must carry his accoutrements, arms, cartridge, etc., aggregating in some armies as much as 70 pounds. When, besides, defective or poor food, impure water, exposure, etc., and other frequent accompaniments of a campaign are taken into account, one need not wonder that disease is a far greater factor as a cause of debility and death than wounds.

"Briefly, fatigue should be considered, owing to its inhibiting influence on the adrenals and the immunizing process in which they take part, as an important predisposing cause of disease. The periods of rest should be so adjusted, therefore, as to counteract this by far the most destructive factor of active warfare. In civil life, such hardships are seldom endured, but here likewise much could be done to prevent infection by means calculated to insure the functional integrity of the adrenals.

"To stimulate the adrenal functions when marked fatigue prevails would, of course, only aggravate the hypoadrenia after perhaps a period of temporary betterment. The powdered adrenal substance should, on the other hand, judging from the effects of injections of adrenal extracts in experimentally fatigued animals, serve a useful purpose."

I always correct my patients when they call our treatment a "stimulation" of the adrenal gland. We assure them that it is a regeneration of the gland, not a stimulation. Drugs may be used to stimulate the adrenal, but as Dr. Sajous assures us, such treatment can offer only a short period of "temporary betterment" followed by an aggravation of the hypoadrenia. It is for this reason that the medical profession has so much trouble treating CFS. The word "regeneration" does not seem to be in their lexicon.

In this last paragraph Dr. Sajous also recommended taking powdered adrenal substance. To show that there is nothing necessarily new under the sun, this substance, properly prepared so as not to lose any of its natural factors, still remains the backbone of our treatment of CFS today. The work of this pioneering endocrinologist can never be sufficiently appreciated. We can only thank God for his great insight and candor and attempt to carry forth the work he began. It is only sad to see how few of his own compatriots have had the incentive and wisdom to follow his lead.

Expanding Understanding of the Disease

A few years after Dr. Sajous' initial work, Henry R. Harrower, M.D., F.R.S.M. (London), in his book, *Practical Organic Therapy, The Internal Secretions in General Practice*,[2] asserted:

"Since the adrenals are so extremely susceptible to so many outside influences, it is likely that they would be easily worn out, and as a matter of fact, 'functional hypoadrenia' is as common a condition as any endocrine manifestation. From a practical standpoint, this is an extremely important symptom complex."

This was written a short time after World War I! Dr. Harrower continued:

"It is quite some years since Sajous began to emphasize the importance of this condition, and while his opinions were scorned, and some of his ideas declared visionary, it must be admitted that our present knowledge of this subject is very much in harmony with the following quotation from Sajous' monumental work: 'Functional hypoadrenia is the symptom-complex of deficient activity of the adrenals due to inadequate development, exhaustion by fatigue, senile degeneration, or any other factor which without provoking of organic lesions in the organs or their nerve paths, is capable of reducing their secretory activity. Asthenia, sensitiveness to cold and cold extremities, hypotension, weak cardiac action and pulse and anorexia, anemia, slow metabolism, constipation, psychoasthenia are the main symptoms of this condition.' "

---

[2]Harrower, Henry R. *Practical Organic Therapy, The Internal Secretions in General Practice*, 3rd ed. Glendale, CA, The Harrower Laboratory, 1922.

Harrower went on to say:

"Asthenia is the rule and muscular tone (both striped and unstriped muscles) is poor. Exertion is impossible and the fatigue syndrome is prominent. The intestinal musculature is inactive and stasis, a common cause of hypoadrenalism, is also a usual result of it. Mental exertion, even the simplest exertion, often causes so much weariness and exhaustion as to be prohibitive. Mental elasticity is lost, and there is both mental and physical depression with the fear that the individuals now cannot accomplish their accustomed good mental work; and the story that they 'have lost their nerve.' With this, one frequently notes a fearfulness of making wrong decisions and vacillating and indecisive frame of mind. This is the most usual form of adrenal insufficiency. It is chronic both in origin and in its course."

Another section in Harrower's book is entitled "Neurasthenia as an Adrenal Syndrome."[3] The word "neurasthenia" is not used as much today as it once was, nor is it as well understood by the general public as it was at one time. Neurasthenia means weak nerves. Although they may not have heard of neurasthenia, people frequently speak of their weak or sensitive nerves and upset nervous system. I personally still find neurasthenia an acceptable term and an exact description of many patients I see daily. My own feeling is that most of the so-called neurasthenia of old was plain old (or should I say new) CFS.

Again, Harrower's report was so lucid that I include here the entire section on "Neurasthenia as an Adrenal Syndrome":

"The minor form of 'functional hypoadrenia' is more common than some have appreciated, and the fact that there is a psychic origin as well as the other physiologic causes already considered, allies it to the fashionable neurasthenia of today. In fact, some have stated that what is improperly called

---

[3]Since it seemed most appropriate, "Adrenal Syndrome" was the term I used for Chronic Fatigue Syndrome until the latter name became very popular. I still think the Harrower term is more informative and descriptive.

'neurasthenia' is not a disease per se, but really a symptom-complex of ductless glandular origin and that the adrenals are probably the most important factors in its causation. Campbell, Smith, Osborne, Williams, and others, including the writer, have directed attention to the importance of the adrenal origin of neurasthenia (though a pluriglandular dyscrasia is practically always discoverable), but so far this is not understood as well as its frequency and importance warrant.

"A few quotations from the literature will firmly establish the importance of this angle from which to study this common and annoying symptom-complex. Quoting from the Journal of the A.M.A. (Dec. 18, 1915): 'The typical neurotic generally has, if not always, disturbance of the suprarenal glands on the side of insufficiency. The blood pressure in these neurasthenic patients is almost always low for the individuals and their circulation is poor. A vasomotor paralysis, often present, allows chillings, flushings, cold, or burning hands and feet, drowsiness when the patient is up, wakefulness on lying down and hence insomnia. There may be more or less tingling or numbness of the extremities.'

"...Kinnier Wilson in...'The Clinical Importance of the Sympathetic Nervous System' makes the following pertinent remarks: 'Many of the common symptoms of neurasthenia and hysteria are patently of sympathetic origin. Who of us has not seen the typical irregular blotches appear on the skin of the neck and face as the neurasthenic patient works himself up into a state'? The clammy hand, flushed or pallid features, dilated pupils, the innumerable paresthesias (tinglings), the unwonted sensations in head or body, are surely of sympathetic parentage. In not a few cases of neurasthenia, symptoms of this class are the chief or only manifestations of the disease. Here, then, is a condition of defective sympatheticotonus; may it not have been caused by impairment of function of the chromophil system [adrenal system]?...There does not appear to me any tenable distinction between the asthenia of Addison's Disease and the asthenia of neurasthenia. Cases of the former are not infrequently diagnosed as ordinary neurasthenia at first. It is difficult to avoid the conclusion that defect of glandular function is responsible for much of the clinical picture of neurasthenia...[Wilson] makes the following apothegm: 'Sympathetic tone is dependent on adrenal support, and until the glandular equilibrium is once more attained, sympathetic symptoms are likely to occur.' "

Interestingly, the 1915 quotation from the *Journal of the American Medical Association* postulated a relationship between neurasthenia and low adrenal function. Yet to this day, such a relationship is rarely considered in medical treatment. At our Healing Research Centers, we consider such cause and effect to be very common and we treat it accordingly. Undoubtedly, because of this, we have become internationally known for our treatment of the weakened nervous system.

The most important advances in endocrinology made by Dr. Harrower were in connection with what he called the "plural glandular treatment." In this form of treatment, he found it far more efficacious to use a variety of glandular substances than to use a single one in attempting to correct this or any of the glandular imbalances. In preparations he himself made and marketed, he, for instance, combined thyroid, pituitary and sex-hormone substances along with what he called "remineralization" techniques, that is, the use of certain mineral elements plus his adrenal-gland substance to treat "Adrenal Syndrome." Such plural glandular technique is used to this day. With modern methods of tissue-nutrition analysis, however, we are able to individualize the therapy for the specific case at hand to a far greater degree than was possible in Dr. Harrower's day.

While Dr. Sajous brought the condition of functional hypoadrenalism to light, described its symptoms, illustrated some of its causes and suggested certain types of therapy, the further development of this therapy was in the hands of Dr. Henry Harrower. Dr. Harrower's work, however, was little appreciated by his contemporaries, and although he was able to help thousands of individuals during his lifetime, he was never able to convince more than a handful of his medical colleagues of the value of the plural-glandular substance therapy. Since this therapy was based on supporting nutritionally the glandular components of the body, the results, though definite and long-lasting, were slow in developing. This fact probably led the medical profession to disregard them in favor of the quicker-acting (but noncurative) single-hormone preparations and synthetic compounds.

It is important to make a distinction between the use of endocrine hormones and endocrine substances. Even these early investigators realized that if the body is given a hormone which is produced by an endocrine gland, the gland, due to the natural functioning of the body's homeostatic mechanism, will stop producing its own hormone as long as the external hormone is being supplied. If this process is carried out long enough, the gland involved will actually atrophy, and eventually it stops producing hormones. If, on the other hand, a patient is given glandular substance that is free from hormones but contains the other nutrient elements of the gland intact, this substance acts as a food to build and regenerate the gland, so that it may once again be able to regain proper functioning on its own. This is the basic difference in theory and practice between the medical practice of endocrinology and the natural or nonmedical practice of endocrinology. These early researchers realized that except in emergencies, nutritional glandular therapy was the only practical, physiological way of reestablishing normal function among the endocrine glands. In emergencies, it may be essential to give pure individual hormones for a short time, but these should be exchanged for the glandular substance therapy as soon as possible.

Of course, if the involved gland has been destroyed and there is no hope of regeneration, it may be necessary to give hormonal agents for life. However, this is not the case in most chronic glandular deficiencies such as CFS, and the use of single hormones (such as cortisol derivatives) is usually to be avoided except in a true emergency. We spend a great deal of time and energy working our CFS patients off of such medication that they have been put on by medical practitioners who do not understand the nature of this condition.

While on the subject of glandular substance therapy, I need to warn our readers that all glandular materials are not the same. As the use of these products has become increasingly popular, many unqualified producers have sprung up to supply the demand. Some of these are only out to "make a buck" and have little comprehension of the processes required to make a therapeutically effective preparation. In earlier editions of this book, we recommended several trade name products that we found effective in treating CFS, but we will not do so in this edition. The reason for this change is twofold: (1) New and sometimes better products are being produced at an accelerated pace now that our work is becoming better and better known and (2) some of our old standbys have not kept up with advances made in nutritional science and may no longer be the state-of-the-art they were when we first wrote this text. Therefore, we will discuss generic remedies in this edition, but will not suggest specific manufacturers. For specific products we invite you to call us at 1-800-300-5168. In this way we will always be able to give the names of state-of-the-art glandulars and other remedies needed to treat CFS.

Continuing Research

The work of Dr. Sajous and Dr. Harrower has been continued by a small group of medical practitioners, one of the most dynamic of whom is John W. Tintera, M.D. In 1955 Tintera reported on the hypoadrenocortical state and its management, and in 1966 he advanced the hypothesis that reactive hypoglycemia may result more from hypoadrenocorticism with deficient counterregulatory responses of the adrenal cortex than from insulin excess.[4-5] (A later study on hypogly-

---

[4]Tintera, John W. The hypoadrenocortical state and its management. *New York State Journal of Medicine* 55:1869, 1955.

[5]Tintera, John W. Stabilizing homeostasis in the recovered alcoholic through endocrine therapy: Evaluation of the hypoglycernic factor. *Journal of the American Geriatrics Society* 6:126, 1966.

cemia in insulin-dependent diabetic patients acknowledged indeed that deficiency in counterregulatory hormonal responses is important in hypoglycemia reactions[6]).

Tintera described, in lay terms, the functional insufficiency of the adrenal glands in an article in *Woman's Day* in February 1959, entitled "What You Should Know about Your Glands and Allergies"[7]:

"Think of your adrenal glands as the two central command posts, one perched above each kidney from which your body's chemical defenses are mobilized and directed. Think of pollens, house dusts, and all other allergy-producing substances as attacking invaders (which they are, of course). Now you're right up against the basic and real reason why many people suffer from allergies while some people hardly know what the word means.

"What happens when the central command posts of allergic bodies fail to command the chemical defenders? Attacking invaders are on the ramparts, but the defenses are enfeebled and disorganized. The invaders get in and bring about the damage which results in wheezes and sneezes, sniffles, hives, rashes, skin eruptions, and other miseries and also sets the body up, chemically, for endless repetition of the same.

"This new knowledge was discovered and proved by endocrinology, that branch of medical science devoted to the study of the body regulating system of internally secreting glands, the endocrines, of which the adrenals are kings. Until endocrinology came up with the all-important knowledge, no one knew the basic cause of allergies."

Rightly, Dr. Tintera said that until recently there was no real, lasting cure for allergies—only temporary relief which often required heroic measures. Usual treatments for allergies and infections were aimed at body chemistry disturbances at

---

[6]Polonsky, Kenneth, and others. Relation of counterregulatory responses to hypoglycernia in type I diabetes. *New England Journal of Medicine* 307 (18):1106 1112, October 28, 1982.

[7]Tintera, John W. What you should know about your glands and allergies. *Woman's Day* February 1959, pp. 28-29, 92.

or near the surface. He continues as follows:

"Actually, many allergies are only the end results of processes that have their beginnings in adrenal gland failure. Most people stand up well against attacking invaders—so well that they do not know they're under attack. But 17,500,000 Americans [almost 10 percent of the population] succumb so readily to the same invaders they know only too well they are being attacked!

"Endocrinology has now gotten deep down below the end results of allergy processes. In learning about the intricate and subtle chemistry of the adrenal glands, it discovered that the difference between the non-allergic majority was the difference between strong, alertly responsive adrenals which can and do marshal the body's defenses in a flash, and weak, sluggish glands which are incapable of doing what they should.

"I'm an endocrinologist. In more than 20 years of a busy practice with thousands of patients, I've yet to work with an allergic patient whose troubles weren't basically due to his poorly functioning adrenals, or who wasn't relieved of his allergic woes when his adrenals were put into proper working order. Included among these patients were sufferers of asthma as well as of hay fever, people 'sensitive' to beef protein as well as those 'sensitive' to house dust or to tomatoes or parsnips or whatever the so-called 'sensitizing agent' happened to be."

To Tintera there are not "kinds" of allergies, only one "kind"—impaired adrenal glands. For many years before this glandular basic cause was discovered, it was held that allergic persons were allergic to many substances—not just one. He found the identity of the "sensitizing agents" of little more than academic interest because the controlling and only important matter is the state of the central command posts of bodily defenses, the adrenals. He continued:

"In understanding why this is so, let's begin with the fact that body chemistry is exceedingly intolerant of all substances not strictly its own. Foreign substances, for the most part, are broken down and converted chemically; animal proteins into human proteins, vegetable carbohydrates into human carbohydrates, etc.

"But there are many foreign substances which body chemistry can't handle by conversion. Some have to be neutralized chemically and so made harmless, and these are the 'allergens' which cause allergies if neutralization doesn't come about. Others have to be killed or at least prevented from multiplying, and these are the living bacteria which cause infections if body chemistry fails to deal with them.

"Taking ragweed pollen, for example, the pollen gets into the body through nostrils or mouth and burrows into nasal membranes. It cannot be dislodged by mucous flow or by sneezing, and it cannot be absorbed through conversion into a compatible chemical. If something isn't done, there will be inflammation and swelling of membranes of indefinite duration as more and more pollen gets in.

"So there is an emergency. The alarm runs along nerveways to the cores of the adrenals (the 'medulla,' in medical parlance). They respond by secreting a chemical or hormone. The blood carries it to heart, lungs, and other glands of the endocrine system, and back to the adrenal casings, the 'cortex' ... The medulla hormone stimulates lungs into providing added oxygen, heart into producing a faster blood flow, and the cortex into secreting a host of hormones which first call forth the neutralizing chemicals from various body cells, then put them together in assorted ways, and finally command their assault on the attacking invaders. All this happens in a flash. The amounts of chemicals involved are so very tiny they're hardly measurable. The increases in heart and lung actions are not enough for the mind to be aware of them. Just the same, a highly successful defensive operation has taken place. Definitely the body in which it happened is not allergic."

This defense, he asserted, takes place no matter where the attack occurs—in the membranes of the bronchial passages, the stomach lining, or the skin.

"The principal defensive weapon on the battlefront of surface membrane is the 'antibody.' For successful defenses there must be antibodies for every variety of disease-causing bacteria or viruses; specific antibodies for pollen, for house dusts, tomatoes or parsnips, or whatever the foreign substance which is both inert and foreign and, therefore, is an 'allergen.'

"The amazing thing is that the antibody for any given invader cannot exist until the invader actually attacks. Body chemistry takes the invader's chemical measurements, so to speak, and proceeds to tailor an antibody which fits the invader to a 'T'. This intricate, fast-moving chemistry takes place in the spaces between cells which are bathed in the body fluid called lymph. Lymph has chemical interchanges with the blood through the lymph channels and those channels have way stations or depots, the lymph nodes.

"In the nodes, from materials fetched through the channels, are manufactured floating cells, lymphocytes, which first collect the newly-formed antibodies and then carry them to the membranes where the invaders, having caused the antibodies to be formed in the first place, are digging in. Now, we are at the key point. Antibodies cannot be formed and the lymphocytes cannot discharge their burdens of antibodies without the assistance of the hormones of the adrenal cortex. If the adrenal cortices are underfunctioning, if they are semi-exhausted and unable to respond fully to stimulation, these essential hormones are either insufficient in amounts or they are chemically out of balance. Here, then, is the basic cause of allergies and infections."

Dr. Tintera explained that the cortex of the adrenal secretes no fewer than thirty-two hormones (we now know of several more) when functioning healthily. They and the hormones of the medulla are so vital in body chemistry that without them life is impossible.

"Routinely they regulate the chemical conversion of our food into both fuel and building materials; they regulate the transport of the fuel throughout the body for 'burning' with oxygen in each and every tissue, and the transport of the building materials and its uses in repairing and replacing old cells and tissues. On the emergency level, adrenal hormones prepare the body to withstand stress of whatever kind and degree."

Regarding stress, he wrote, "Walking is stress because it burns more body fuel. Running is a greater stress and so are heated arguments, tearful, and other powerful emotions, and thousands of other things which require changes in blood flow rate, in the diameters of arteries and veins, in the tensions of muscles....

"All these stresses are perfectly normal and it is no less normal for our bodies to be under constant attack by 'foreign' invaders since everything outside ourselves is foreign. But this constant attack is constant stress. Add everything together and you get the idea of how much work our adrenals are required to do. They are uncomplaining strong organs when all is well with them, *but some people are born with undersized or weak adrenals, due to the accidents of heredity.* [Emphasis added.] Under the stress and strains of living, the question for any individual is how much his adrenals can take; how much reserve strength...they have.

"A person with very poor adrenals may never be affected by it if he lives a completely sheltered life, free of extraordinary stress. But that kind of life is neither desirable nor possible. Stress is the essence of living; from it comes pleasure and happiness. But if the adrenals are not thoroughly competent, each stressful incident cuts into their reserves. The day must come when those reserves are exhausted and the whole body is in trouble.

"That explains why some people are allergic and susceptible to infections from birth while others are adults before those calamities befall them. One had poor adrenals from birth and the other had adrenals without enough reserves to last. And you can almost be positive that in any of these cases, the built-in weakness has been compounded many times by the common American diet which is bad enough to pull down even the strongest adrenals."

Dr. Tintera asserts that the adrenals in all his allergic patients are weak and semiexhausted, secreting their hormones in insufficient and unbalanced amounts. His treatment to cure them of their allergies is an injection of an extract of beef adrenals which contains the whole assortment of adrenal hormones in the balance drawn up by Nature. This permits the beaten-down glands of the patient to rest by adding hormones to body chemistry that take over the work. He does not use cortisone or its derivatives except in emergencies because, to be successful, the drug must be given in amounts that would upset the balances between the different groups of secreted adrenal hormones and would cause adrenal atrophy if given over a protracted period. His patients were required to follow a high-protein, medium-fat, and low-carbohydrate diet. This permitted all meats and fish, all dairy products, all fruits, and all vegetables, except the very starchy ones. It forbade all stimulating drinks, especially alcoholic ones. This diet was designed to place the least possible stress on the adrenal glands, thereby permitting them to function at top efficiency. This diet does not exhaust, but rather builds, adrenal reserves. Fortunately for all CFS sufferers, our adrenal glands have great recuperative power; they will again be our willing servants if we but give them the chance.

We can see from Dr. Tintera's work that not only is the Adrenal Syndrome problem flourishing today, but it is actually much more pronounced than it was in the times of Sajous and Harrower. Why? Simple. Its causes are becoming more and more pronounced on all levels of our daily life with the continued assaults to our body by more and more sophisticated drugs and medicines and continued assaults from the outside due to increasing forms of pollution, contamination and toxicity. The wonder is not that there are people who are affected by CFS; the real wonder is that there is anyone in the country who does not have this condition. It is amazing that any of us is able to function in a truly normal fashion and adapt to the great number of stresses and general assaults to our body, mind and soul that abound today.

Dr. Tintera's work also reveals new aspects of the adrenal gland, particularly its control of allergies. Most patients who have allergies are victims of CFS even though they do not as yet have the other classic symptoms. Dr. Tintera's comment on inherited adrenal weakness is also interesting. My work has consistently verified this point, and I now refer to these patients as having "Chronic, CFS."

Current Concepts

Despite all the recent concern about CFS relatively little has been done in recent years to explore and clarify the biochemical alterations in the body which cause this condition. One research study that reviewed the relationships between adrenocortical function and infectious illness stressed the presence of depressed adrenocortical secretion during chronic infection, although most information was based on studies of tuberculosis.[8]

Perhaps the most exciting and promising advance toward understanding clinical disorders and illnesses brought about by early delicate hormonal imbalances has been in the realm of thyroid physiology.[9-13] This research has been concerned with relationships between hormonal secretions and depression. In studies of depressed patients, testing with the hor-

---

[8]Rapoport, M. I., and Beisel, W. R. Inter-relations between adrenocortical functions and infectious illness. *New England Journal of Medicine* 280(10):541 -546, May 6, 1969.

[9]Prange, A.J., and others. Effects of thyrotropin-releasing hormone in depression. *Lancet* 2:999-1002, 1972.

[10]Loosen, Peter T., and Prange, Arthur J., Jr. Serum thryotropin response to thyrotropin-releasing hormone in psychiatric patients: A review. *American Journal of Psychiairy* 139(4):405-416, April 1982.

[11]Gold, Mark S., and others. Grades of thyroid failure in 100 depressed and anergic psychiatric inpatients. *American Journal of Psychiatry* 138(2):253-255, February 1981.

[12]Gold, Mark S., and others. Hypothyroidism and depression: Evidence from complete thyroid function evaluation. *Journal of the American Medical Association* 245(19):1919-1922, May 15, 1981.

[13]Amsterdam, Jay, and others. Thyrotropin-releasing hormone's mood-elevating effects in depressed patients, anorectic patients, and normal volunteers. *American Journal of Psychiatry* 138(L):115-118, January 1981.

mones was the only early method of detecting hypothyroidism, as results of usual laboratory tests remained in the normal range. This research is exciting, because revelations in this area may provide clues which will lead to better understanding of CFS—not only its causes, but the disease process as well.

Meanwhile, Dr. Hans Selye, the Canadian physiologist, in his long-term study of stress and its effect on the human body developed a theory he called "General Adaptive Syndrome" (GAS).[14-15] According to Dr. Selye (see his chart in Chapter Five), the body contains a complex mechanism designed to permit it to adapt continually to the various stresses and pressures that assault it from all sides, inwardly and outwardly. As long as this system is capable of functioning in a more or less normal fashion, the human body and mind are able to adapt successfully to a wide range of stresses and assaults, whatever their nature—chemical, physical, bacteriological, viral, mental, or emotional.

"Actually, this ability to adapt is common to all forms of life. When a life form can no longer adapt, it becomes extinct. In other words, this ability to adapt is the very essence of life itself. The mechanisms in the human body which produce this adaptation are, admittedly, complex and, as yet, not fully understood, but one of the most important entities in this adaptation is the adrenal gland. Without this small but mighty gland sitting like a bishop's cap on the top of the kidney, we would not be capable of adaptation. With a strong and vital adrenal gland, we are capable of adapting to almost everything Nature and life can throw at us. With a weakened or poorly functioning adrenal gland, the ability to adapt becomes more and more difficult until a point is reached at which it is difficult for an individual to function productively in our stress-filled, high adaptability-requiring society."—Hans Selye.

Because of the central position of this gland in Dr. Selye's

[14]Selye, Hans. General adaptation syndrome and diseases of adaptation. *Journal of Clinical Endocrinology and Metabolism* 6:117-230, 1946.

[15]Selye, Hans. *The Stress of Life.* New York, McGraw-Hill Book Company, Inc., 1956.

General Adaptive Syndrome, I originally called Chronic Fatigue Syndrome, which basically is a poorly functioning ability to adapt, Adrenal Syndrome (taking it, as mentioned before, from the works of Dr. Harrower). The name was short and descriptive, though certainly not all-inclusive. As previously mentioned, it should not be confused with other presently known conditions, except possibly Addison's disease; but, since this latter condition is caused by distinct pathology of the adrenal gland, differentiation should be easy. Henceforth in this book, when I speak of Chronic Fatigue Syndrome (no longer Adrenal Syndrome), I refer to that condition of the neurohormonal system that produces a weakening or breakdown in the body's general adaptive mechanism.

The whole theory behind the adrenal gland as the culprit (or is it the victim?) in CFS can be stated simply if we take into consideration the previous discussion. There is within the body a mechanism that controls: (1) tissue repair and regeneration, (2) one's ability to fend off substances that might cause allergic or similar reactions in the body, (3) one's ability to withstand stress and to be capable of meeting the needs of the environment at any specific time, and (4) the prevention and overcoming of all forms of disease. It is this system that animates and vitalizes us to become vibrant, useful members of society. As long as this system functions normally, there are few problems of life, be they physical, mental, or emotional, which we cannot overcome. It is the great productive center of all strength and vitality in the body. No matter what difficulties the body may encounter, as long as this adaptive mechanism is functioning well, we have every opportunity to overcome these problems. If there is a weakening or a breakdown in this system, everything else in life falters. Every molehill which the average person would leap with ease becomes an insurmountable mountain to the individual with CFS. The simplest of life's tasks becomes complicated and monumental when the general adaptive mechanism is not up to par. At first the mind still functions and ambition is alive, but the body is not capable of carrying out the directions of these motivators.

Eventually, frustration develops which causes depression, further exhaustion occurs due to stress and worry, and finally even ambition and mental capabilities themselves come under the influence of this weakened system. In extreme cases, suicide is not unknown among the victims of this disorder. There have even been reports of Dr. Jack Kevorkian (the death doctor) helping CFS patients to attain what is to them the final cure.

While the history of the condition now known as CFS is long, there is every reason for hope for the CFS patient. The proper treatment is safe and sure if the patient can but understand and accept the true nature of this condition. Once this is accomplished then he has only to follow our instructions, and his adrenal glands can begin their journey back to strength and vigor.

Summary

Functional Hypoadrenia, Adrenal Syndrome or Chronic Fatigue Syndrome, a condition of the neurohormonal system, produces a weakening in the body's ability to respond to stress and if not arrested can lead to a breakdown of the body's ability to function. Until recently this condition was not easily diagnosed. In fact, for most of its existence diagnosis of this condition was usually accomplished only by a process of exclusion. Although CFS under various names has been recognized for more than a century, it has changed little in symptom pattern and in treatment required to help it until recently. I personally feel that the "chickens" of infant multiple immunizations, overuse of man-made drugs, suppression of natural disease processes by antibiotics, increased pesticides and other toxic substances in our environment "have come home to roost" and the result is an exponential increase in this weakened adrenal syndrome.

At the turn of the century, Charles E. de M. Sajous, M.D., pioneered in the study and the treatment of adrenal gland malfunction, citing fatigue and other bodily abuses as major causative agents. He understood this condition so well that the admonitions he gave to his patients are still the backbone of the life-style we recommend for all our CFS patients. Although we may be able to refine his suggestions to make his admonitions more specific and sophisticated for a more rapid and complete recovery, the basis of all CFS treatment was outlined long ago by this intrepid pioneer.

Henry H. Harrower, M.D., in the period following World War I made advances in treatment of adrenal malfunction, using what he called plural-glandular treatment—a treatment still used today in our Healing Centers.

John W. Tintera, M.D., continued studying functional adrenal disease, especially the relationship of adrenal malfunction to allergens.

Another doctor who made an important contribution to this subject is Hans Selye, Ph.D. He identified the General Adaptive Syndrome theory, describing it as the mechanism by which the body adapts to various stresses and pressures by controlling tissue repair and regeneration, fending off substances which might cause allergic or similar reactions, withstanding stress, being capable of meeting the needs of the environment at any time, and preventing or overcoming all forms of disease. In CFS, the general adaptive mechanism is unable to perform these functions.

In our own more than four decades of working with CFS, we have discovered that the malfunction of the adrenal gland results from a negative interaction of heredity, stresses of all sorts and a combination of individual symptoms or idiosyncracies.

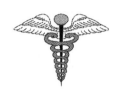

Chapter Three

The Nature of the Patient

(The first part of this chapter is taken from the 1983 book *Adrenal Syndrome*. My original intention was to completely rewrite this chapter, but as I read and reread it, I decided to leave it as it was and add new material to bring it up-to-date. While the 1983 text seems a little naive today, the basic underlying principles are still the same we consider today.)

N my original 1975 publication on the Adrenal Syndrome, I described the nature of the adrenal patient thusly:

Before discussing the treatment of hypoadrenalism used at our Clinic, let's consider the nature of the person who is most likely to develop this disorder and the manner in which it is produced. If I could describe the hypoadrenal patient in one single word, that word would be "sensitive." He is cognizant of all that is going on around him, and he feels an overconscientious sense of responsibility about those near and dear to him and even about the whole world. This person's nervous and glandular systems are delicately balanced; yet he is willing to take the cares of the world on his own shoulders.

Such a nature is not sufficient alone to cause adrenal insufficiency. In my own estimation, a hereditary weakness of adrenal structure must be present. There are some persons who fit this description but who nevertheless have sufficient glandular vitality to avoid adrenal hypofunction. On the other hand, we do find persons who are by nature not perfectionists or inclined to drive themselves, yet suffer from this ailment. In these persons, it seems that the hereditary weakness is so strong that even a relatively normal amount of stress is sufficient to cause adrenal hypofunction.

Differences in Degree of Symptomatology

Not counting various external, physical, bacteriological and chemical stresses, the two basic causes of Chronic Fatigue Syndrome (CFS) are unremitting stress on an individual and the degree of hereditary weakness in the basic neurohormonal system on which the general adaptive mechanism depends. The CFS patient is a combination of these two factors. These factors can be in any proportion and the variation in this proportion produces the different reactions shown by various CFS patients. For instance, a patient may have only a mildly weakened general adaptive system, but be subjected to severe and unremitting stress in his life. If so, there is a good chance that eventually the general adaptive system will break down. This patient is a CFS case and in need of treatment; however, the character and extent of his problem are different from that of the individual who has a severe hereditary or congenital weakness in his system and in whom seemingly insignificant stresses can produce severe CFS difficulties. Both patients require treatment and much of the treatment is similar, but the emotional counseling and the general tenor of the psychological approaches to these two patients are entirely different.

The degree of symptomatology in a patient can often be

calculated as a sum of these two factors. On a hypothetical scale of one to ten, taking one as normal and ten as severe, the first individual might have a two on the hereditary scale, but a nine on the stress scale. Together they total eleven. On the other hand, the second patient may have a two on the stress scale, but a nine on the hereditary scale. Together they also total eleven. The severity of symptoms in these two would be similar because of the eleven reading, but treatment would vary because of the different causes.

Obviously, the person who registers one on both scales has little problem. If a person rates a five on both scales, he approaches the area of symptoms. As patients display greater hereditary weakness and stress, say a seven on one scale and an eight on the other, they are going to have larger problems. In assessing the nature of the adrenal patient, these two interdependent factors which produce CFS must be considered.

All CFS patients are scored on these two scales for degree of hereditary weakness and degree of stress, and the doctor who treats them must ascertain their score on each scale as accurately as possible in order to prescribe the proper treatment so they may return to normal.

CFS patients should be divided into two separate groups. First, that group which I stressed in my earlier work who, although they have certain hereditary weaknesses, are basically normal human beings who have been subjected to various stresses which have caused a definite, demonstrable change in their general adaptive systems. Second, those patients, and unfortunately their number is large, who have such defective general adaptive systems that the ordinary and mundane stresses of life leave them exhausted and incapable of coping. The latter patients require the most understanding and the best treatment we can give. They require the full understanding and cooperation of their families and friends. They generally require lifelong treatment of one sort or another to help keep the general adaptive system in a reasonable form of functioning activity. There are no factors in their lives that can be ignored. There are no thought processes in their minds that do not affect for good or ill their basic problem, and, yes, their entire existences. It is really for this group of individuals that this book was written. The first type of CFS patients can gain adequate information for their needs from my original text, but for those sufferers whom I now call chronic Chronic Fatigue Syndrome patients, the first work (1975 edition of *It's Only Natural*) was only an introduction. For them, a complete commitment on the part of themselves, their families, their friends and their doctors is absolutely necessary for a proper resolution of their problem.

It is true that stress is not what happens to us, but how we react to what happens to us. This statement must be qualified, however. When a CFS patient has advanced to a certain stage in his condition, his mind, due to a variety of difficulties the two most important of which are lack of oxygen to the brain and cerebral allergies, cannot properly evaluate the stresses under which he is placed. The patient's mind simply is not capable of reasoning to the extent necessary to prevent further damage to the general adaptive system. It is necessary that patients in this condition be placed in an environment which is as stress-free as is possible and given proper treatment until improved cerebral activity allows them once again to be able to regulate and evaluate the stresses of their own environment. These patients, usually those with strong heredity factors, are so overwhelmed by common stresses that life in an ordinary household becomes almost untenable until some improvement in their condition is made. The nature of emotional stress in the individual with a weakened adrenal system can be so complex and so incomprehensible to the average person that he often may seem mentally disturbed. No other group of people more exemplifies the truth of Benjamin Franklin's statement, "*Those who have nothing to bother them will be bothered by nothing,*" than do those with CFS. With a weakened adrenal mechanism, the tiniest molehill becomes a Mount Everest. The slightest misconstrued remark becomes condemnation of a major magnitude. The most sedentary physical task is an insurmountable obstacle.

Example of Hypoadrenalism

Hypoadrenalism commonly occurs in a person who has cared for a loved one through a long, extended illness. Take, for instance, a woman whose husband developed cancer and was operated on unsuccessfully. Physicians gave up all hope, but the man had a sturdy constitution and lived on for a year or so before he finally succumbed. The family, not wealthy, could not hire nurses and others to care for him, so his wife took care of him. She often was up day and night, watching out for his needs. The man she loved for many years gradually changed. Little by little he withered before her eyes. His emotional nature changed and he became a most difficult person with whom to live. There were times she wanted to scream at him, yet she knew that would not be kind or socially acceptable, so she held it in. She could not get her proper rest. She did not eat properly because she had lost her appetite. Instead she snacked on foods that did not supply her body with the vital elements she especially needed at the time. Her adrenal glands, willing servants that they are, kept pouring out hormones to sustain her during the entire time. Unfortunately, they, like her, got little respite.

The unremitting and constant stress intensified. Although the glands can recuperate during sleep to some degree, her rest was less than normal and her glands had little time for their own regeneration. But they are valiant friends; they did not give in. They kept functioning and working well beyond their normal requirements.

Finally, death came to the husband. But stress was not over for the wife. She had to deal with the undertaker and then the lawyers. Then the government, inconsiderate relatives, and other people disturbed and even preyed on the recent widow.

During all this additional stress, her steadfast adrenal glands kept working their best to produce the substances she needed to keep going. Finally, she was able to rest. The undertaker, the relatives, the lawyers, and even the government were satisfied. At last she could relax. What about her

47

adrenal glands? They were exhausted. They, too, demanded a well-earned rest. As soon as the stresses were removed and the adrenal glands were not needed to the extent they had been during heavy stress, their function slowed to enable regeneration for the preservation of the whole physical system. The widow suddenly felt tired and exhausted. Expectably, she went into a period of depression and exhaustion.

Depending on the basic hereditary integrity of the adrenal glands, at this point she might or might not develop hypoadrenalism. If the glands were basically strong and healthy, she would be able to recuperate and pick up her life in a reasonable time. If the glands were inherently weak, she might develop hypoadrenalism. If the glands were weak, when they became so exhausted, even with the rest they were receiving, they might not be capable of regeneration to their normal state. They still were functioning, or the woman would die, but at a level far lower than before the prolonged period of stress, much lower than the level needed for normal daily existence.

We have just reproduced a classic case of functional hypoadrenalism (now called CFS). Although there are many other ways of describing this syndrome, from this case history certain specifics can be derived about the nature of the stress most likely to produce this condition.

First, although the stress itself is not necessarily great, it is generally unremitting. Also, we sensitive humans are not able to overcome it—either because of a sense of responsibility or because of our emotional dependency. That is, even though it was exhausting her adrenal glands, the wife in the above example had no choice but to take care of her husband. For her own physical well-being, she could have abandoned him, turned him over to relatives if such existed, or tried to get the state to take care of him. It would have prevented her from developing hypoadrenalism, but her own sense of responsibility would not have allowed it. In my experience, I have found most stresses that produce hypoadrenalism come from doing what a person believes to be his duty. If we are to prevent hypoadrenalism in those who are susceptible, we must teach them to learn to control their response to the stress.

Our attitude—what I call acceptance of the stress—is often on par with or even more important than the stress itself in producing reaction. For example, had the woman whose husband was dying been able to rearrange her life, much of her later trouble could have been prevented. She could have eaten foods and nutrients that are best able to build up the adrenal glands, supporting the glands through this difficult period. With more knowledge she could have changed her basic attitude toward her husband at this time to a complete acceptance of his condition and of his unavoidable death.

From the foregoing, one can readily see how easy it is to develop CFS. The situation described is all too common, but the patient should be capable of responding within a fairly short time if she is receptive and if adequate treatment is given. The problem with so many cases is that only rarely is treatment given toward rebuilding the general adaptive system. The patient is usually untreated and must live through the ensuing years as best she can. Much of her ability to improve depends on the stresses placed upon her and upon the basic integrity of her general adaptive system. If her future stresses are within reason and her adaptive system relatively normal, she may gradually return to a normal state of health and productivity, time and rest being a good doctor in this instance. On the other hand, if her adaptive system is marginal and the stresses of widowhood difficult, without specific treatment she may never return to normal and may even continue to deteriorate with time. If such patients would seek the help of professionals trained to intervene in this condition, much misery and nonproductiveness could be prevented. It would be interesting to take a survey to find out how many on our ever-growing state and federal welfare rolls are actually victims of this disorder. The normal mind and body is a productive mechanism. It is designed as such and likes to work as such. When it does not, one certainly has the right to wonder if it is functioning normally or whether it is in some unknown manner defective. Are the so-called poor really lazy and hereditarily unproductive, or are they perhaps victims in many cases of a dysfunctional adaptive system?

"Chronic" CFS

How do individuals with "chronic" CFS differ from patients with the simpler type? How can you as a husband tell if your wife has this problem? How can you as a mother tell if your son or daughter is a chronic CFS sufferer? How can you as a lover tell if your future mate may have this difficulty? The answers are not easy, but there are answers.

Differences in Types of CFS

When I first interview a patient, I look into his eyes. We are told the eyes are the windows of the soul. That may be true, but they are also the windows of the general adaptive system. Persons with chronic CFS show to a lesser or greater degree an appearance in the eyes that is unmistakable to the trained observer. They have a certain vague staring, a vacantness which in my experience is without precedent in other disease conditions. It is nearly impossible to describe, but the person who has seen it once will never miss it again. A similar appearance is found in those who are taking street drugs and in some who imbibe too much alcohol, but while similar, there is a distinct difference between the look of the chronic CFS patient and those who have been taking drugs or alcohol.

When these patients are examined, a difference in their blood pressure levels between the reclining and the standing positions is often registered. In general, the blood pressure is somewhat lower than normal in these patients and tends to drop, or at least not to rise as it should in normal individuals when they stand up from a reclining position. For instance, if a normal blood pressure reading is 120 over 80, chronic CFS patients may have a blood pressure reading of 110 over 70 in the reclining position, but when they stand, it may drop to 100 over 70 or even to 90 over 70. The amount of the drop is usually indicative of the severity of the condition. There are many qualifications concerning this testing mechanism, however. If a patient with chronic CFS constantly attempts to force himself to activity, he may show the same rising of blood pressures when he stands up as do normal individuals. However, after waiting a minute or so, the blood pressures will gradually start to drop because his adrenals are simply not strong enough to hold the higher level for any length of time. In my earlier book, I stated that the amount of drop in the postural blood pressure is indicative of the condition of the adrenal patient. This is still true, but as suggested here, must be interpreted with many reservations. One has to know how to read these pressures and equate them with the nature and the state of the patient at the time of the reading. Of recent years I have come to use the expression of the eyes as far more indicative of the state of these chronic adrenal individuals than the postural blood pressure readings, although the latter are still of great value, especially if they include the resting pressure, the pressure immediately upon standing, and the pressure at 20-second intervals for a minute to a minute and a half while the patient remains standing. The amount of drop and the speed of drop as time progresses give a good indication of the state of adrenal functioning.

In regard to postural blood pressures, a patient may come in feeling exhausted and yet have a good blood pressure reading. On the other hand, a patient may come in feeling quite well with a poor blood pressure reading. This may be explained by the fact that there is always a certain time lag between the exhaustion of the glands and the symptoms produced; blood pressure usually predicts how patients are going to feel rather than how they are feeling at that time. For instance, if a patient who is feeling poorly has a good pressure reading, I can usually predict with confidence that he will improve within a day or two and feel much better. On the other hand, if a patient feels good but has a poor reading, I usually advise that patient to increase his medication and to take it easy for the next few days or he will go into a period of decline.

Further information necessary to diagnose the chronic CFS case must come from the patient's history. This history usually shows that the adrenal patient has had spells of exhaustion, weakness, inability to concentrate, poor memory, allergic sensitivities, sensitiveness to many ordinary situations and so on as far back as he can remember. Most often these victims started to notice their difficulties at puberty, although many assure me that they had the symptoms even earlier. There is a group which did not notice difficulties at puberty, but did notice them in their late high school years or when they tried to keep up with the rest of the students in college. In this latter group, most went away to college, lived in a dormitory or apartment, did not get sufficient sleep, ate poorly—either insufficient amounts or junk foods or both, had stressful relationships with members of the opposite sex, may or may not have had financial difficulties, and were overconscientious in their studies, often attempting to obtain grades that were beyond their native abilities. These stresses are exactly the type to trigger a latent chronic CFS.

Other histories show that the first signs of this syndrome occurred shortly after marriage or after the births of children. All of these events have this in common: They are normal stresses of existence which occur at various times in our lives and which our adaptive mechanism should take in stride, but which are sufficiently stressful in individuals with a weak adaptive system to trigger the full chronic CFS. This hereditary weakness must be compared to an internal bomb that only requires sufficient stress to act as the spark to light the fuse, and once it is set off, one's system is, like Humpty-Dumpty, difficult to put back together again.

The character and mechanism of a chronic adrenal case can generally be differentiated from the hyperstress-type case because the chronic patient shows symptoms at an earlier age, though not invariably so, but more importantly, tends to be triggered by stresses the average person should be able to handle without real difficulty. This last factor is the true dividing line between these two types of CFS patients.

Symptoms Similar to Mental Illness

Most chronic CFS patients are considered by their friends, relatives and health practitioners—the people from whom they seek aid—to be suffering from some form of mental or psychological disturbance.[1] This is true to such an extent that during our first interview with them, the majority of these patients assert they are sure that they have mental or psychological problems. One of the first and most important tasks of our therapy is to convince them that this is not true. Unless we accomplish this, treatment is difficult and sometimes nearly impossible. Many of these patients are called schizophrenic, some paranoiac, some manic-depressive, and most are called neurotic. This is not to say that all schizophrenic, manic-depressive, or paranoid patients are merely chronic CFS victims. There are true paranoids, true schizophrenics, and true manic-depressives, but chronic CFS can mimic the symptom patterns of all of these mental conditions. What I am saying is that any person, who has been diagnosed as having one of these conditions should be examined to also determine whether possibly his condition is chronic CFS. Such patients are brought almost daily to our Clinic. Many are helped because, as it turns out, they are suffering from chronic CFS, and therefore can be treated by specific physical means.

Determining Characteristics

From among our thousands of patients we have found a variety of interesting characteristics which are of great help in understanding and diagnosing CFS. A history of these might be helpful to those who are themselves wondering whether they or one of their loved ones might have this ambiguous but disabling disorder.

---

[1]This is much less true today than when it was written in 1983. More and more doctors are accepting the concept of the CFS patient. However, it is sometimes difficult to convince the patient and his family that there is not some form of mental disorder. As many patients have stated to me, "There sure are times when I feel crazy."

"Don't Make Me Wait!"

It is difficult for these people to wait calmly for any length of time. Usually either one of two things happens when they attempt to wait. Either they gradually become more and more exhausted until they simply have to lie down and rest, or they gradually grow irritable to the point that they become extremely disagreeable,[2] ready to lash out at almost anybody about anything. In our Clinic, I specifically tell all chronic adrenal patients that when they have to wait and feel either of these symptoms starting to come upon them, they are to let the nurse know that they can no longer wait and go to rest or enter some activity to relieve their anxiety. We then call them when a treatment room is available.

When an adrenal patient starts to feel this type of anxiety, he must take action, *i.e.*, remove himself from the environment that is causing the anxiety, no matter where he may be. To sit and fight these sensations is to create more stress and tension, and what is worse, this inaction can produce a destructive, martyred attitude. He might think: "Why does the doctor make *ME* wait?? If he is truly concerned about me, he would not make me sit here; poor little me." This attitude is common and understandable in CFS patients, but it is unproductive and generally unfounded. These patients need only the freedom and the good sense to excuse themselves and to go somewhere to rest whenever this exhaustive irritation overcomes them.

Sometimes if I am not specifically sure of the diagnosis of a difficult case, I may let the patient sit in my waiting room for

---

[2]We now know that patients who react in this fashion are in what Dr. Hans Selye called the "Countershock Phase" or the "Resistance Phase" of CFS (see Chapter Five). In this phase the Hypothalamic–Pituitary Axis attempts to overstimulate the adrenal gland to make up for the gland's weakness. Admittedly this is like whipping an old tired horse. Eventually, as shown clearly in the Selye chart, these patients will advance to the final "Exhaustion Phase" if they are not treated properly. Patients in this stage now make up the bulk of our new CFS patients and usually their previous treatment only exacerbated the situation; but more on these patients later.

some time, observing him repeatedly out of the corner of my eye for signs and symptoms of either of these states. If either of these patterns occurs, I can be pretty sure that a diagnosis of chronic CFS is accurate.[3]

"You Make Me Mad!"

One somewhat common experience of these patients that had me befuddled for a while was finally clarified in my own mind by a clinic case. The patient, the wife of a judge in a southwestern state, was an obvious chronic CFS victim who had been placed on heavy doses of amphetamines for many years to keep her functioning. Even with these, however, she awakened in the morning feeling so exhausted and depressed that she had little desire to get up or to attempt any activity of the day. She had discovered, however, in some accidental way that if she became angry, gradually she would start feeling better and eventually be able to get up and go about her daily duties. While she was staying at our Clinic, she vented her imaginary wrath on the first person she saw in the morning. This was usually a member of the kitchen staff bringing her breakfast. This anger was quite vehement, as extreme emotion was necessary to stimulate her poor, abused adrenals to even a modicum of activity. Of course, this daily occurrence was soon reported to me. Whenever I visited this patient a little later in the morning, she always was in a very pleasant and good humor, as the wrath had dissipated as soon as the adrenals were stimulated. I could not understand what the kitchen staff had complained about. Only later, after the patient had left our Clinic, was I able to consider the situation calmly and understand the mechanism behind her early-morning tirades. In this particular instance, the taking of amphetamines for a long period of time had created such a constant stimulus to the adrenal system that even they were no

---

[3] With our new tests, especially the Adrenal Stress Index (ASI), we no longer have a need to use such measures to confirm the diagnosis of CFS, but this reaction on the part of a patient is still very indicative of the condition.

longer adequate to get her glands started after a night's rest. It took the strong stimulus of rage to wake up her poor, weakened adrenal mechanism. The problem with this method of adrenal stimulation was that the degree of rage necessary to get her going created severe stress on everyone around her. While this patient was at our Clinic, our staff absorbed the force of her conduct, but when she returned home, her husband was the sole recipient. Little wonder that he was so anxious to have her remain with us!

While this was certainly the most extreme case we encountered of anger being used to activate the system of a chronic adrenal patient, this same action occurs to a lesser degree in many victims of this disorder. I have as patients many women with this problem who, when the stresses get too great, throw themselves into a state of severe hysteria and remain in this state until they have sufficiently stimulated their adrenal system and poured sufficient hormones into their bloodstream. While this method may give a short-term burst of energy, it is short-lived and is always followed by greater adrenal weakness.

"But I Just Can't Forget It!"

Another common characteristic of chronic CFS is the patient's inability to clear the memory of consciousness of personal problems so that treatment and cure can proceed. Probably because of poor circulation and therefore poor oxygenation that is common to the brain of these patients, the normal reasoning faculties, particularly those used to distinguish between that which is rational and that which is not, do not function as they should. Therefore, these patients have difficulty clearing their minds of certain thought processes which unfortunately remain imbedded, as it were, in the memory and constantly act as recurring stresses which make treatment most difficult. Possibly some specific form of chemical activity due to a failure of the general adaptive system allows this to occur in the brain. In the near future we may be able to ascertain this chemical activity, and by neutralizing it hasten the patient's ability to free himself from these retained unproductive thought patterns.[4]

A few simple examples illustrate this point. In an unguarded moment, a husband may have said something to a wife that she misunderstood and he did not fully mean. The normal wife can rationalize after a while from his actions that he really did not mean what he said and then forget it. The chronic CFS patient often cannot free the incident from her consciousness. She constantly turns it over and over in her mind, building stress to the point that she cannot sleep, and at times may go into fits of uncontrolled anger and hysteria. Counseling, even by the best of physicians, often has little effect on these patients. About the only help at the present time for this patient is an active treatment of the general adaptive system to improve the oxygen-carrying power to the tissues of the brain so that it can again function in a more rational manner. This will usually work, although it takes time to clear some patients' minds, and the unfortunate obsession can be very painful and trying to those who are near and dear to these patients.

Or, for example, because of a patient's gradual deterioration into chronic CFS her husband may no longer think of her as desirable. He wants a divorce. She is told that the only way of preventing this is to once again make herself desirable. The way that this must be done is to cure her chronic CFS. However, the fear of losing her husband becomes such a chronic stress that it makes therapy difficult. As rapidly as treatment strengthens her general adaptive mechanism, she tears it down by worry and concern over a situation which can only be corrected by the treatment which she is negating by her actions.

---

[4]Since this was written there has been a great deal of research into methods of helping this problem, and many have proven helpful to some patients. In our own experience the best method to overcome this difficulty is to regenerate the adrenal gland by our usual procedures of both active and passive adrenal treatment. As the glands become more normal, so do the mental abilities.

Both of these cases illustrate what I mean when I say that this condition is self-perpetuating and "feeds upon itself." It produces emotional patterns that by their nature tend to worsen the condition itself. These states I have called the "dead-end canyons of emotions," in that while the emotion exists, it creates nothing productive. All it can do is tear down and destroy the basic functioning of the body.

Summary

Chronic CFS patients have a condition that is basically a general adaptive system weakness. Their bodies cannot adapt to the stresses placed upon them. In the group of patients with the milder form of CFS, the body may be basically normal, but the stresses placed upon it are of such a magnitude that it starts to malfunction, at least temporarily. Treatment usually corrects these cases fairly quickly, and as long as the patients are somewhat careful of future stresses, they can usually avoid returning to the CFS.

For the vast number of people who have an inherent hereditary weakness of this adaptive mechanism, knowledgeable and extensive treatment is usually required over a long period of time, but they can be returned to life as functioning, productive members of society. To achieve this end takes true understanding on the part of their physicians, their families, and their friends, and, to some degree, from society as a whole.

Relationships with Others

Mother–Daughter Relationship

Many CFS patients show a strong hereditary influence that usually can be directly related to one parent or the other. The most common relationship that I have found in our clinic is the mother–daughter inheritance. A woman who has a CFS problem may have sons who exhibit the problem, but almost inevitably her daughters will have a tendency to CFS. Conversely, when I see a young woman with CFS, inevitably, on checking, I find that her mother has or has had a similar problem. The inheritance may come through the father or may, as mentioned, affect male offspring. But the invariableness of the mother–daughter inheritance is worth mentioning here. When we encounter a CFS patient, we also make an effort to influence other members of the family to be checked for the condition. This is of great importance should a young mother exhibit the syndrome. While her children may be too young to show symptoms, we know from experience that unless their neurohormonal mechanisms are strengthened, they will undoubtedly have trouble as they approach puberty. In these instances, we try to institute minimal basic treatment at an early age to forestall the nearly assured development of CFS in these young children. This is particularly important in the case of daughters.

Relationships that Strengthen or Weaken Patients

Certain types of individuals help to strengthen adrenal patients, and certain types tend to weaken them. This susceptibility to individuals may vary greatly, depending on the state of health of the CFS patient. Much of this has to do with the personality of the friend. Full of animal magnetism, some people have a surplus of energy and goodwill. The chronic CFS patient absorbs from these persons and benefits thereby. But the relative or friend must be careful to not allow the adrenal patient to absorb so much energy that he—the relative or friend—is left depleted of his own needed energy.

Some people are "emotional vampires," so devoid of energy and love within themselves that they attempt to sap others whenever possible. If a CFS patient gets into the clutches of one of these individuals, he can be drained of his remaining vitality in short order. In general, if a patient feels stronger after being with a person, well and good. But if the patient always feels worse, beware, for that person might be an enervating entity, an emotional vampire.

Those with a predilection to chronic CFS, seemingly by a natural selective process, usually marry an individual who is at the opposite pole of neurohormonal integrity—which is a scientific way of saying that a woman, who is delicate and weak in the neurohormonal system, by nature invariably marries a man who is strong and solid in his neurohormonal makeup. It is almost as if when she was young she knew that it would take a man of such qualities to watch over and protect her through the difficulties possible in the ensuing years. Often these individuals have little in common, but in the long run they need one another to fulfill specific purposes in their lives, and so the marriages are generally successful, at least as far as permanence is concerned. I have known a few CFS patients who married one another. The results were usually disastrous because of the instability of the chronic adrenal individual. Somewhere in the life of a CFS patient there has to be a rock-stable person to offer support and sustenance, or his whole existence is built on constantly shifting sands.

An individual with CFS can often help another patient, especially in the early stages, by letting him know that he is not alone with his unfortunate problem. One of the most common symptoms of the chronic CFS patient is a feeling that he has an illness that no one can understand and that no one has had before. Friends and relatives assure him that they have never heard of anything like it. This is, of course, because so few doctors acknowledge the condition and so little publicity has been given to it.[5]

Mixed Vibrations

Many individuals who are drained of energy by those around them feel that they are victims of agoraphobia, that is, fear of crowds, mainly because when they are in a crowd, they

---

[5] This has now changed, but not necessarily for the better. There is now much publicity, but most of it is not particularly helpful. CFS patients have gathered themselves into support groups, but in our experience most of these are mainly "pity parties" that do little to elevate the consciousness of the individuals involved. All too often these groups are filled with a negativeness that tends to pull down the level of all to the lowest of the patients participating.

find that they grow weak and anxious. Generally this is not true agoraphobia, but merely the draining effect, or what I call the "leeching effect," that crowds have on CFS patients. This is one of the earliest symptom patterns I usually notice in CFS cases. Years ago when I first started to practice in Seattle, Washington, a patient who had been a lifelong music lover stated that within the last year she had enjoyed concerts less and less. It seemed that each time she went to a concert, she became exhausted and quite agitated. Upon examination, she was found to have a relatively mild adrenal weakness, and with proper therapy was able to regain her health soon and fully enjoy her love of music once again.

Many CFS patients are sensitive to the mixed vibrations of any large group of people. Each human being is a radio transmitter sending out a vast number of different frequencies which create a so-called "aura" or emanation about him. With most of us, our own vibrations are so strong that those of other people around us have only a minimal effect. To the truly sensitive hypoadrenal victim, however, this effect can be powerful, even to the point of leeching his very energy. His own vibrations can be so weak that he readily absorbs the vibrations and emanations that come from other people. Because of this effect, CFS patients must be careful with whom they associate. On one hand, they find that association with certain persons tends to strengthen them as long as the liaison is not too long. On the other hand, they discover others who enervate them after a longer or shorter period. It is essential to their progress that they shun individuals who sap their energies. But it is to their benefit to associate with persons with whom they feel an increase in energy.

As the number of persons the CFS patient encounters in a group increases, the chance of benefiting from the association decreases. As the vibrations of more and more persons are present in the atmosphere around the CFS patient, the chances become increasingly great that the mixture of these electromagnetic vibrations will adversely affect the patient. Due to this fact, we usually recommend that these patients stay away from crowds as much as possible.

If there is a function the CFS patient wishes to or must attend, however, we suggest that he remain for as short a time as possible, and even then try to choose such associations as carefully as possible to ensure many beneficial vibrations present. For instance, a patient may wish to go to a concert of classical music, and if it is not too long the patient may gain from the exposure.

The Telephone and CFS

Over the years I have noticed a rather unexpected problem with CFS patients—they can be adversely affected by talking on a telephone, much more than if they had the same conversation in person.

In the early days of the Clymer Health Clinic, we had as a CFS patient a fine older Amish gentleman. During the work week he would improve steadily, but he would be in worse condition every Monday morning following Sunday, when he was not treated. At first I thought that he was just missing the treatments on Sunday, but this schedule did not seem to bother the rest of our CFS patients. In attempting to find the answer to this conundrum, I sat him down one day and had him tell me just what he did do with his Sundays at our Clinic. "Well," he said, "since there is not much to do here on Sunday, I usually call all my friends at home on the telephone." That, I felt, was my answer.

I asked him to help me with an experiment. I wanted to have him refrain from doing any telephoning the next Sunday so we could see if this had anything to do with his Monday morning weakness. He thought I was crazy but agreed to follow my suggestion. The next Monday morning he was better with none of the weakness he had been experiencing in the past. This convinced even him and so he rarely made any more phone calls and was soon good enough to be released.

While there is no scientific research I know of to back me up, I feel it is the restricted frequency range of the telephone receiver that affects my CFS patients. We know, for instance, that restricted light frequencies can have a serious detrimental effect on the pituitary and other endocrine glands, so why could not the restriction of audio impulses on the ear and auditory mechanism have a similar stress effect on the glandular system?

Even Happiness Hurts

One characteristic of the neurohormonal exhaustion produced by CFS that is different from the type of exhaustion produced by any other condition is that even events and circumstances that the patient enjoys or that might be a happy surprise fatigue and weaken him. For the patient who loved chamber music concerts they were a great joy, and yet they created sufficient stress, because of the people involved, to be detrimental to her neurohormonal system. Almost all other forms of depression, anxiety, tension, and so on are improved by happiness and pleasant events. A surprise birthday party, a visit from a long-forgotten friend, or a telephone call from a sweetheart—all of these things strengthen the body and spirit of almost everyone except the CFS patient. This is perhaps the saddest component of the entire condition, but it is nevertheless pathognomonic of the disease. When an individual becomes exhausted or physically weakened by events which most people consider pleasure-producing and uplifting, you usually can be sure that this individual is suffering from CFS.

Summary

No two CFS patients have like conditions or react similarly to treatment, because of differences in their heredity and stress. The disorder, it has been noted, most often passes from mother to daughter. A more severe appearance of the condition called chronic CFS may be recognized by a vacuity or glassiness of a patient's eyes and by extremely low blood pressure readings when the patient stands. Patients with chronic CFS as a rule become agitated if they have to wait, may go to great lengths emotionally in order to "awaken" adrenal function, and are unable to forget negative incidents. For CFS patients, relationships with others are often debilitating. Crowds have a negative effect. They should spend little time on the telephone, since it usually has a deleterious effect on them. Persons with chronic CFS don't react positively to surprises; they find that some friends weaken them, others strengthen them.

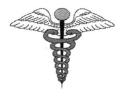

Chapter Four

Patient and Family Responsibilities

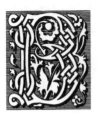Y its inherent nature, Chronic Fatigue Syndrome (CFS) requires more patient cooperation and responsibility in its mastering and cure than any other medical condition known to me. Undoubtedly, this is one of the major reasons why it was so long ignored by the medical community, and why even today most physicians who do recognize it still assure their patients that there is no viable curative treatment. And from their point of view this may be true. There is no magic silver bullet they can give the patient to cure him of this agonizing affliction. The physician, no matter how accomplished, cannot cure CFS by himself. All honest treatment of CFS requires a great deal of work and dedication on the part of the physician, the patient, and especially those around the patient, both friends and family. In my experience, few practitioners are willing to spend the necessary time and effort to program, manage and constantly encourage the CFS patient so that he is capable of carrying out his own part of the cure.

Only the CFS patient himself can obtain ultimate mastery of his condition. The physician must provide a certain segment of the treatment. His part is essential and vital, but by itself is not sufficient for the total correction of the ailment. Full recovery from CFS is possible only if the patient assumes his part of the responsibility. If he does not, all help will be slow, arduous, and eventually incomplete.

If this book succeeds only in helping the myriads of patients who suffer from CFS to successfully understand the nature of this condition and their personal responsibility in its correction, it will have fulfilled one of its main purposes. Prior to the issuance of *Chronic Fatigue Unmasked,* all that was available to help the CFS patient was the twenty-seven page chapter on stress and hypoadrenalism in our first book, *It's Only Natural* All new CFS patients in our Clinic were told to read that chapter two or three times before their next appointment. I felt that was the only way they could achieve any semblance of understanding of their situation so that I would be able to help them. This understanding is still an absolute essential for patient care. For current CFS patients, we insist they read this text. Whenever they feel depressed or have doubts about their condition, I encourage them to read and reread the exposition of CFS as given in this chapter.

Steps in the Patient's Recovery

There are five important steps which the patient must take to help himself in overcoming this condition:

> 1. The patient must fully understand the character and nature of CFS.

> 2. The patient must accept the fact that he is a victim of CFS; not only must he accept this fact in his mind, but also in his heart and soul, so that he has no doubt at all that this is the problem and that he must face it squarely if he is going to conquer it.

> 3. The patient must evaluate his entire lifestyle in light of his CFS.

> 4. The patient must correct his previous lifestyle so that he can produce the amount of stress reduction that is required in his specific phase of the CFS.

> 5. The patient must realize the necessity of, and embark upon, a program of stress reduction

that will continue the rest of his life.

Step 1: Understanding the Problem

Everything a patient does in his life—be it working, resting, exercising, sleeping, eating, enjoying entertainment, taking part in any form of activity—helps either to strengthen or to weaken the adrenal glands, thereby either helping or exacerbating his CFS. Therefore, it is imperative that the patient know as much as possible about the nature of every factor, variation or nuance that might affect him on the road to recovery. My own crusade, which now extends over four decades, has been to investigate each and every physical, mental and emotional facet of life that may in some way or another help support or injure my patients' adrenal function. You will find the results of this dedicated effort between the covers of this book.

Each bit of understanding and information the patient can glean about his problem increases his chance for a more rapid and uncomplicated recovery. If questions and doubts arise, the patient is able to return to this text to search for an answer. If a patient has a thorough understanding of his condition as presented here, he should meet few situations in his existence which he cannot understand and explain. Doubt, fear and depression arise more from not understanding the real nature of the condition than from any other single factor of CFS. If a patient has a set of disturbing symptoms, but knows what bodily function is not operating properly and what has caused the malfunction, together with what he must do to alleviate it, a great amount of stress and worry is prevented, and treatment of the condition can progress unhindered. On the other hand, if a patient is having difficulties which he cannot explain or understand, thoughts start passing through his mind that the difficulty might be this disease or that disease; these fears create stresses which produce more symptoms which lead the patient further down a destructive path and can create a serious setback to the improvement of his condition.

The first step on the road to recovery from CFS, therefore,

is to understand and comprehend the basic adrenal reactions in the various phases of the condition as outlined in the chart of Dr. Selye. Unfortunately, this is a step ignored by all too many patients. A good baseball coach always spends a great deal of time acquainting his players with the basics of the game, for he knows that in the long run this knowledge usually means the difference between success or failure. Such instruction often seems dull to the new players since they want to get out on to the playing field, but the coach knows such basics are the only road to real accomplishment and that the player that is not well-grounded in them will never be a good athlete. So it is with the average CFS patient. He wants to get started with his treatments and does not want to be bothered with all this talk about his phase and what he must know and do to assure his improvement. But just as with the baseball player, if he is deficient in the basics, he will not be able to meet the challenges of the various phases of his condition as they arise. The best advice I can give patients is to return to this text and read and reread it until the fundamental nature of the condition and its various phases is well understood and its various ramifications and nuances become as well known as the letters of the alphabet.

It is not always easy for the CFS patient to comprehend his condition as readily as a more stable person might, because by nature CFS causes mental clouding, poor concentration, and inferior memory retention. Therefore, it is necessary for the CFS patient to spend much more time going over this knowledge to absorb it, but with persistence he will always succeed. For those who have difficulty with the written word, they may be better able to absorb the instruction if someone else will read it to them. This will help the reader, a close friend or relative we trust, to better understand the patient as well.

Step 2: Accept the Condition

Step one, patient understanding and comprehension, is relatively easy to explain to the patient and the instructions for its fulfillment are rarely misunderstood. Unfortunately, this cannot be said of step two: patient acceptance of the condition. This point can present a hurdle that can be the most difficult part in the entire treatment of CFS.

For treatment of CFS to proceed as quickly and as fully as possible, it is vitally important that the patient direct all his energies toward helping himself to overcome the difficulty. The only way that we can help him marshal these energies is if he is positive about what is wrong with him, if he accepts this fact fully, and therefore is completely motivated to help the doctor overcome his malady. Unless this can be done, recovery will be unnecessarily slow and probably incomplete. Recovery from CFS always proceeds in direct proportion to the amount of patient acceptance achieved.

If the above statements are true—as they are—and assuming that the average patient is at least reasonably intelligent, one might readily ask why we have so much trouble obtaining patient acceptance. If this acceptance is essential for the well-being of the patient, why cannot the patient recognize this and do all that is necessary to help the doctor aid him in his recovery from this condition?

To understand the patient's difficulty, let us reconsider the nature of the condition, the nature of the CFS patient and the advice of the various physicians the patient may have consulted before us. In past years, most of these patients had been diagnosed as neurotic or just plain lazy. But they know that something is really wrong with them, and so most have fears that some strange, undiscovered disease is gradually eating away at their vitals. Even the diagnosis of CFS is of no great help, since once this diagnosis is made, they are told in the next breath, "There is no known cure for your condition." Strangely, these patients are often relieved when they develop a treatable condition, even a serious one. Just yesterday, one of my CFS patients told me how she startled a surgeon, who had just told her she had breast cancer, by saying, "Boy, am I glad that's all it is, I was afraid it might be another manifestation of CFS." "After all," as she asserted to me, "they do have a treatment for breast cancer."

When the symptoms of the condition are under control, it is easy for a patient to be logical and reasonable and accept the possibility that he may have CFS. However, when in the still of the night some of the more bizarre symptoms of this condition occur, it is extremely easy for fear and apprehension to creep into the patient's consciousness or for words of a physician who once pronounced him emotionally unstable to come vividly to mind. Doubt builds on doubt, and by morning the patient can have himself thoroughly convinced that he is mentally unstable or a victim of some undiscovered incurable disease.

On the opposite side of the ledger, it is difficult for individuals whose symptoms are not as severe as some others to accept the fact that they have a condition as complicated as CFS. They want to believe either that they are only overworked or that all they have is some undiscovered virus.

Step 3: Evaluate

If he expects to really improve, it is necessary for the CFS patient to go on a true austerity program as far as the expenditure of his own neurohormonal energies is concerned. If he is able to adjust his life-style to conserve these energies as much as possible, he will be able to rebuild the general adaptive mechanism and "pay up" his past bodily debts. When these are paid off and the neurohormonal mechanism is brought to a state of optimal functioning for this individual patient, his austerity program, *i.e.*, his life-style, can be liberalized to a maintenance schedule. However, he must be careful that he does not once again overextend himself and produce more debts—the practice that had previously brought him into such a poor state.

All patients ask, "Just how much must I adjust my life-style?" The answer is at once simple and immeasurably complex. They must adjust their life-style sufficiently to produce the necessary stress reduction of the neurohormonal system to allow it to regenerate and return to normal. Exactly what this means for any individual patient depends on three factors:

First, on the extent of the drain on the neurohormonal system; second, on the present life-style of the patient; and third, on the types of treatment the patient is able to obtain for his condition. Only after analyzing these three elements are we able to help the patient in the evaluation of his life-style changes.

For example, I once had a young minister from Pittsburgh as a CFS patient. His condition had become so severe that he had fainted in the pulpit while delivering a sermon. This reaction, not all that uncommon in CFS patients, occurred because his low blood pressure delivered a deficient amount of oxygen to his brain. At other times, he had became so weak that he had to spend two or three days flat on his back in bed before he could carry on with his work. He was, however, as are so many CFS patients, a definite overachiever. As soon as he was able to get out of bed, he was out working on church duties, giving lectures in different parts of the country, attending parishioners and planning new projects. Since he lived about six hours from our Clinic, it was not possible for us to see him frequently, so every attempt was made to find a physician in his local area who was knowledgeable about CFS. As previously reported, those who would accept him as a patient seemed to have little knowledge of CFS, and those who were knowledgeable refused to accept him as a patient. Since clinical treatment of any significant magnitude seemed out of the question for this patient, a radical change of his life-style was essential if improvement were to be obtained. He had to give up as many of his external church duties as possible and delegate wherever possible his internal church duties. Eventually, once he was able to regenerate his system, he could gradually return to his various duties. However, I do not believe that even under the best circumstances he should ever return to the full intensity of activities he was fulfilling when I first saw him. Admittedly, such an opinion is not what a patient wants to hear. In fact, this patient has had a difficult time accepting our diagnosis of CFS. Nature has a way of helping truth, however, and once he again fainted during

71

church services, he had little choice but to accept the condition.

In another case, a patient called on me, describing in great detail all her symptoms, each one of which led to the same conclusion—CFS. She mentioned that while she wanted to come to our Clinic for treatment, it was going to be difficult for her, because she was at that time holding down three jobs and was working seven days a week. I remarked that her situation would probably be quite easy to help; all she had to do was to give up at least one of her jobs and use that free time to come to see us at the Clinic. I advised her that, in fact, unless she did so, there was probably little that I or anyone could do to help her overcome her CFS.

Another patient whom I had been treating for some time achieved good progress at first, but could not progress beyond a certain plateau. Review of her treatment program showed she was receiving all of the remedies, following the proper diet, and getting her proper treatments at the Clinic. Only one thing remained for her to do: Change her life-style sufficiently to reduce stress further because she was, as I had told her, still putting out more energy every week than she was producing, and therefore creating an ever-increasing debt rather than building up a reserve in her energy bank. I learned later that she had been active in certain church activities which, while she enjoyed them, were not an absolutely essential part of her life. Once we were able to convince her to give up these activities, within two weeks she started to improve again and was able to continue that improvement. Eventually, as her neurohormonal mechanism strengthens, she can again include these extra church activities in her life. However, had we not analyzed her life-style and changed it at the time we did, she would undoubtedly still be floundering in her recovery and wondering why she did not make the improvement we had promised her.

Step 4: Reduce Stress

Once the patient has adequately evaluated his life-style, he can correct his way of living and begin the accomplishment of stress reduction. In regard to this point, one is constantly reminded of the familiar Biblical phrase, "The spirit is willing, but the flesh is weak." It is one thing for a patient to evaluate his life-style and realize what changes must be made, quite another for him to institute these changes and maintain the changes until proper improvement has been attained. For instance, the young Pittsburgh minister, while obviously aware of the measures necessary for alleviation and correction of his problem, was anything but eager to make those changes and was actually strongly opposed to them. Well motivated to work for his ideals and life objectives, he had a strong sense of duty and responsibility to those who were dependent on him. He was willing to make almost any sacrifice except that which would entail a change in his basic life-style. In fact, his resistance was such that he altered his life-style only when his symptoms became so severe that he could not physically continue. This is not unusual. In fact, just as I was writing this paragraph, I had a phone call from a Jewish CFS patient who told me she could not come for treatment next week because the treatments make her tired for a couple of days (they shut off the adrenal gland so it can regenerate) and her religious holidays are coming, and she wants to prepare for them. We only trust that the delay in treatment and her added committed stress will not set her progress back too much.

A long-time professional acquaintance of mine, Dr. Henry Linke, often said "The way a patient has lived is what has caused the problem he now has. To help the problem, we must change his life-style. You cannot ultimately do one without the other." Dr. Linke told me that over forty-five years ago, and each passing year has reaffirmed the truth of his statement.

These first four points of patient responsibility are obviously interdependent. Before a patient is able to change his life-style, he must understand his condition, and therefore have a reason to change. People do not make changes without a reason or purpose. Once a patient understands his condition, it is easier to accept the difficulty and realize the only way to overcome it is to make the necessary changes in his life-style. He must then, with the aid of a knowledgeable physician, plan these changes, and again with the help of his doctor, carry out the alterations that are essential to his ultimate recovery.

Step 5: Continue the Stress-Reduction Program

Once changes have been instituted and the patient is on the road to recovery, he must consider establishing within himself a never-ending evaluation of the stresses to which he is exposed. Stress is an integral component of life without which life would be nearly valueless. The various stresses of living prompt us to all forms of activity which produce every known improvement and man-made beauty in the world about us. In some individuals, however, an overabundance of stresses can exhaust their neurohormonal mechanism. CFS patients must be careful to avoid an abundance of stress; they must shun those stresses which are by their very nature worthless or useless. We refer to such stresses as worry, anxiety, judgment of others, or paranoid-type fears. These stresses have no redeeming features except that by learning to eliminate them we are able to grow stronger and wiser.

As I write these words I have just received a phone call from one of my CFS patients in France. She is taking a "pain pill" for her fibromyalgia and another drug to help her sleep. She expressed great concern over these drugs and stated that she was "worried to death" that she would not be able to "get off them" and that they would set back her CFS recovery. I told her that I was much more concerned regarding her worrying then about the drugs she was taking. I let her know that her worry would set her back much worse than the effects of the drugs. I told her, "I can help you get off the drugs, but I can't stop you from worrying; that you have to do for yourself."

Probably the most common question asked me by those with CFS is, "Will I ever be normal again?" The answer I give is, "There is no such thing as a 'normal' person. We are all crippled to a lesser or greater degree from birth. We all come into the world with the combined heredity of our mothers' and fathers' ancestors, none of whom were normal, and therefore there is no way that they can create a totally normal child. Your problem happens to be a weakness in the neurohormonal mechanism. Luckily, it is one we understand, one we can control, and in most instances one we can correct. It is necessary, however, for you to live more carefully in regard to the various stresses of life than the individual with a stronger neurohormonal mechanism, somewhat in the same way that the individual who has inherited a mild diabetic condition must watch his diet so that he does not ingest too much sugar. As long as he watches this factor, he can live a relatively normal life. If you, the CFS patient, learn to control and moderate the various stresses upon your whole being, you too can live a relatively "normal" life.

When a CFS patient says he wants to be "normal," he means what he believes is normal. He really does not mean what would be his own normal state, but what he sees as normal for some other person or for the people around him in general. If a blind person is sick and we help him get well, he does not expect to see again, he only expects to have the additional problem corrected. This is not true of most CFS patients. They want us not only to return them to their normal state, but also to make them "see again," *i.e.,* they expect us to help them overcome their congenital neurohormonal weakness. We attempt to do this not by returning these patients to "normal," but by encouraging them to a state of the supernormal. They must work to obtain a greater control over their lives than the average person, for only in this manner may they achieve their desires. My college football team once had a one-eyed quarterback who was good enough to become nationally famous. With his disability, he lacked depth perception, and so had to put forth much greater effort than most to reach his goal. However, he did not bemoan his fate. He persisted, and outpaced all his two-eyed competition for the quarterback position. So must the CFS patient. In the last analysis, how productive, creative, or normal a life the CFS patient lives is entirely up to him. To succeed, he must follow as fully as he can the five tenets laid down in this chapter. He must fully understand his condition, must have a complete acceptance of the condition, must evaluate the stresses upon him and his general life-style, must correct these stresses as necessary, and must be eternally vigilant in evaluating the emotional stresses that may come to him during the rest of his life. He does not need to stay away from all stresses, but all unnecessary stresses should be reduced to a minimum so that his energy can be conserved for those activities and emotional situations that are truly beneficial and productive to him on all planes of his existence.

What Every Family Should Know about the Person with CFS[1]

Almost without exception, the average family and friends of the CFS patient unwittingly do everything they can to intensify the condition. The harder they try to be helpful, the more injurious become the results of their efforts. There are several simple reasons for this paradox, the most common being that almost all intuitive or so-called "gut" reactions toward the CFS victim are invariably incorrect. The advice, be it professional or amateur, given most persons with symptoms similar to those displayed by the CFS patient are completely ineffectual and usually detrimental to the progress of these individuals. Unlike the true neurotic or basic nonachiever, the adrenal victim wants nothing more than to be able to do all the things his friends and relatives are extolling him to do. The fact is, he is physically incapable of accomplishing these tasks and will remain so until the basic underlying condition is remedied.

The patient with this problem is usually intelligent, highly motivated, responsible, with a great desire to achieve. The difficulty is that he has neither the glandular nor the nervous strength to carry out these desires and ambitions. This fact can

---

[1] Also see "A Letter from a Friend Who Suffers with Chronic Fatigue Syndrome" in Appendix III, p. 291.

create in him a large and often conflicting group of emotional and personality frustrations. Put yourself in his place for a moment, and perhaps you will see the degree of frustration that is produced by his condition. You are an individual of intelligence and character. You have desired to do useful and productive things with your life, and yet every time you attempt to do something, you become more and more exhausted. Every attempt at productive activity is met with strange nervous anxieties or, as one patient put it, "agitated depression." The only thing that even remotely seems to help is rest and withdrawal from all the fascinating events of life. You are like an athlete who is trained to run the hundred-yard dash, but who collapses after a few yards each time he attempts to run. Soon you stop trying and wonder if there is any sense in training or in trying to accomplish anything because fatigue, anxiety and failure have become the essence of your existence.

Here, of course, is where your friends and family come to your aid. They entreat you: "Now, come on, don't be lazy. Keep going, keep trying." They tell you: "It's all in your mind. Tell yourself you are going to succeed and you will." You consider that perhaps they are right, and so you try harder. But the harder you try, the more you stress your weakened glandular system and the more rapidly you fail. The more of such admonitions and encouragement you receive from your family and friends, the more guilt you accumulate when you are not able to accomplish what they extol you to do. The greater the guilt, the greater the stress; the greater the stress, the less you can accomplish; the less you accomplish, the more you are admonished; the more you are admonished, the greater the guilt, and so on ad infinitum.

In this way, the most well-meaning friends and family members hasten the development of this disease. In fact, from my many years in treating this condition, I have concluded that the most difficult to resolve and the most prolonged of all stresses imposed on the CFS patient are those placed there by friends and family who are truly trying to be helpful. The ironic saying comes to mind: "With friends like these, who needs enemies?"

In no way do I desire to be critical or unfair regarding the motives of the family and friends of the CFS patient. These patients are the most misunderstood of all disease victims in America today. How can their loved ones comprehend their problems when not even one in a hundred doctors accepts or understands them?

A large part of my time and energy in treating CFS patients is devoted to counseling their family and close friends. Oftentimes only by enlisting their help am I able to resolve a difficult case. When properly motivated, no other group of people can have such a beneficial effect on the victims of this condition.

What Family and Friends Can Do

Understand

The foremost effort that friends can make to help these patients is to understand as thoroughly as possible the nature and character of the disease. To accomplish this end, I suggest that they read this text thoroughly, not just once, but two or three times until the words are engraved on their consciousness and the spirit of the work itself becomes a part of their being as much as it is a part of their afflicted friend's.

There are times, unfortunately frequent in some cases, when CFS patients can be nearly insufferable. At such times it requires the patience and determination of a saint to live with them. Only if the healthy friend or family member is permeated with an understanding of the nature of the CFS experience can he develop the compassion and understanding necessary to help his poor friend or relative on the proper path to improvement and recovery. One who would be of help to these individuals must be able to push aside his own feelings and personal needs as much as possible and learn to say and do those things that are most apt to produce improvement in the sufferer. There are those who are not willing to undertake such a task upon themselves, and many divorces and broken relationships occur because of CFS. Interestingly, as mentioned previously, most persons with chronic CFS tend to marry partners with strong adrenals. This can be true even though the marriage takes place long before real adrenal symptoms manifest. In this way, one partner is steadfast when the other becomes erratic. While such a relationship helps to stabilize a marriage, it does present a problem in that it is difficult for the stronger partner to understand the weaknesses of his or her spouse, since he or she has not experienced similar symptoms. This chapter is intended to help remedy this lack of understanding.

I am often asked: "Doctor, how can I develop this understanding and compassion when the patient seems to do everything he can to upset me?" The answer I give in my office consultations is this: "Suppose you get on a bus and are about to put your token in the meter. Someone enters the bus behind you and steps on your foot while something he is carrying hits you in the shin. Your shin hurts and your foot is sore. You turn around in great anger ready to read the riot act to this inconsiderate, clumsy individual, but upon turning you find that the object which hit your shin was a white cane, the individual you are now addressing is wearing dark glasses and is obviously blind. What happens to your consternation and anger? Immediately, they are brushed aside by a true understanding. You step out of the way and say to the individual, 'Oh, I am sorry, was I in your way? Please let me help you to a seat.' Which you do. Your shin still hurts, your foot is still sore, but your feelings of anger are entirely dissipated and replaced by those of compassion and helpfulness due to the fact that you now have a different understanding of the incident. The events have not changed from the first insult to your body, but your comprehension of what caused the events has changed completely, and so has your attitude. Thus it can and should be with your attitude toward your CFS friend. He is, as it were, emotionally and physiologically blind. He is not able to change many of his actions; he does not hurt you or anyone intentionally. He is driven to these acts by pressures so great, so difficult to control that even a seraph would be sorely tried."

There is a Buddhist saying I am often reminded of in my treatment of CFS patients: "To know all is to forgive all." If we knew and understood what goes on inside the mind of the adrenal patient, we would be better able to forgive him and work to help him on his path back to a productive existence.

Encouragement

Another important step friends and relatives can take to help the CFS patient toward his recovery is to encourage him. One of the basic characteristics of this disease, particularly in its chronic form, is that of discouragement and depression. It seems to the adrenal patient that life is without joy or purpose, that there is no help, and that he is destined to remain forever in the anxious morass of despondency and depression in which he finds himself.

Sermons and admonitions do not help him; encouragement does. Friends should let him know that they understand his problem, that they appreciate his suffering, but that with the proper treatment and care he will improve. They should let him know that although he will have ups and downs—for this is the nature of the condition itself—he must not give up, but must continue his treatment until his efforts are rewarded. There is no end to the value of encouragement for the CFS patient, no end to the need for constant assurance that he is going to get better. In the early stages of treatment, especially for the patient with the chronic form, he has little else to fortify him. His treatment, of course, is helpful, but in the beginning this is directed toward building basic adrenal support and has little effect on his immediate sense of well-being. In fact, early treatment can make the patient feel more tired than previously because the adrenal is rested so as to allow it to regenerate. Encouragement and hope are the mainstay of help at this time. When friends and relatives ask what they can do to help the new CFS patient, I reply that there are three things which they should give in full measure: encouragement, encouragement, and more encouragement.

Reinforcement

"Let Thine Eye Be Single." Another vital factor to which friends can contribute is *treatment reinforcement.* The Bible says: "Let thine eye be single." To succeed, it is necessary to look in one direction, take one way, use one path. Only by directing all his forces and energies along one line can the patient accomplish his goal. This is important in treating all CFS patients, but absolutely essential in chronic patients. Once I have accepted a patient, I attempt to make my treatment plan as clear as possible to friends and relatives close to the patient, so that they can offer their support for this treatment. At no time should the adrenal patient have the slightest doubt that the treatment he is receiving is anything but the best available. Doubt creates negative thoughts, and these thoughts depress the neurohormonal system in such a manner as to make progress difficult.

Because of the lowered blood pressure, and therefore lowered nutrition and oxygen available to the brain of the CFS patient, he has difficulty making decisions and discriminating among types of therapy. He is easily led from one path to another if some outside influence works to move him in that direction. Like all sufferers of chronic diseases, he is hoping for a miracle. There are no miracles in CFS cases, only specific hard work which eventually succeeds in overcoming the condition.

Once a patient has started on a particular plan of treatment, it is incumbent on true friends to help support him in this plan of treatment. The patient should be entreated to continue the chosen treatment plan.

If friends or relatives have any disagreement or apprehension about the type of treatment the patient is receiving, they should discuss this situation with the doctor, never with the patient. If those close to the patient are in disagreement with the treatment, it might be best for the patient to go to another physician. There is little use in a doctor's going all out to help a patient if his efforts are constantly subverted by the patient's friends and family.

In CFS treatment, the doctor must work diligently to build the patient's confidence in the therapy and in the physician's care. Only in this manner will the patient receive the full value of the treatment given. Anything that family and friends do to disturb this confidence can be injurious to the patient and severely slow recovery. I realize very little of this depreciation of the patient's treatment stems from maliciousness or an overt attempt to hurt the doctor-patient relationship. Most of it comes from a sincere but misguided effort to help the patient. Frequently, friends bring the patient newspaper or magazine articles which discuss problems similar to those from which they think the patient is suffering. Usually, these are about conditions that produce symptoms similar to those of the patient's, but that are not related to the patient's own situation. This type of reading produces in the patient who is unwise enough to peruse them a sense of confusion. The patient begins to question his doctor's care and to doubt the benefit of his treatment. This confusion, unless rapidly corrected, may act to eat away at the progress already made and prevent future improvement.

I do not wish to intimate that the therapy outlined in this book is the only possible therapy to help these patients, or that I alone have all the answers for this condition. Patients may be helped in many ways. I have attempted to bring together the best methods I know to form a complete treatment for this most difficult disease. I know that other dedicated doctors also do a good job with these patients, for there are "many ways to skin a cat." However, in skinning a cat, it is best to choose one way and not try two or three simultaneously. Once the patient and his family have chosen a method of therapy, they should stick with it and not confuse the patient by suggesting other doctors or other treatments. Should any treatment not fulfill the doctor's stated goals, the patient has the right to discuss the future with the doctor, and if the prognosis does not seem favorable, that patient may wish to look elsewhere. If the patient or family and/or friends lose confidence in the doctor, another must be sought. While in treatment with any physician, however, the best chance of success for the CFS patient is by full faith in his care. Again, "Let thine eye be single."

Consideration of Other Factors

While the foundation of friends' help to adrenal patients is supported by the three great pillars already mentioned—understanding, encouragement and reinforcement—several other considerations should be mentioned. When a patient's condition is severe enough to require his staying at the Clinic, we usually do all we can to isolate him from stressful influences. Frequently, our main reason for suggesting a patient stay at the Clinic is to remove him from the home environment which aggravates his condition. The patient's efforts to keep in touch with those at home often defeats our treatment plan. The patient sometimes behaves like a narcotic addict in relation to his previous situation. He knows that every time he contacts "the folks at home," they are likely to say things that can trigger old reactions which are detrimental to his recovery. Yet his connection with family and friends is so strong that he continually contacts them even though it devitalizes him both physically and emotionally.

I have found two solutions to this situation. First, I often explain to friends and relatives the character and nature of the condition and what they must do to be of valuable service to their loved one's recovery. Usually this explanation is helpful and sometimes works very well, but frequently family members are unwilling to cooperate or are simply incapable of understanding the situation. In these instances, and in cases in which friends or relatives do not come for consultation, we insist that a patient not contact his friends and relatives until the negative influence can be controlled by the patient's improved physical condition and understanding of his emotional stresses and sensitivities. It is with great reluctance that we impose such a blackout, it being far more advantageous to the patient and to us to have the help and encouragement of those at home, but in many instances we are left with no other alternative.

A Few Precautions

Even when family and friends are understanding, knowledgeable and sympathetic, they should consider a number of important factors involved with patient contact.

All phone conversations should be brief, preferably not over five minutes. Lengthy phone conversations have a deceptively adverse effect on the mechanism of the CFS patient and can exhaust him much more rapidly than face-to-face conversations.

No more than two or three friends and relatives should visit at one time. Most CFS patients are adversely affected by crowds, particularly visitors the patient does not know well or for whom he feels he must put on a "front." Even old friends should not stay too long (an hour is sufficient) to prevent a drain on the CFS patient. A patient may be set back several days in recovery by a visitation of well-meaning friends who wanted to come to "cheer him up." These precautions are most important when the patient first enters the Clinic Sanctuary. However, as the patient improves, such precautions may be relaxed.

I am often asked by persons who sincerely want to help, "What do we talk about with these patients?" Admittedly, this is a difficult point because some patients are very sensitive. If the conversation centers on the patient and his condition, he might feel he is being patronized. On the other hand, if talk is about the things that are going on at home, he may become depressed and despondent because he wishes he could be there to participate, but cannot because of his condition. (Remember, I said that these people are difficult to please.)

A few suggestions may help. First, let the patient talk. Let him tell about the things which are now important to him. What is he finding out about himself and about others? Let him tell about his plans for the future. In other words, take a lead from the patient. If he brings up a subject, discuss it—but carefully watch how he reacts. If he becomes quiet and with-drawn, if his eyes start to look somewhat vague and glassy, he is being exhausted, and it is time to change the subject, or if no improvement occurs with a new subject, time to leave. Visit-ing a chronic adrenal patient is like having lunch with a tiger. It can be done, but it is challenging, and one must constantly be on guard. When the patient's eyes look glassy, it's as if the tiger were swishing his tail; it is time to leave.

Making Decisions

Though difficult, at times it is necessary for the CFS patient to make decisions. To the patient, with his oxygen-poor brain, molehills easily assume the size of mountains. However, certain family affairs sometimes require a decision by the patient. All such situations must be handled with great care and delicacy, for the patient often has difficulty under-standing the exact significance of many of these arrangements. He will frequently lean too far to one side or the other. That is, he may worry unnecessarily over a simple, uncomplicated arrangement in an attempt to make decisions which are not necessarily related to or concerned with the basic problem. Or on the other hand, he may continually ignore an important project which has to be completed within a certain period of time and which requires some decision from him for its completion.

In these situations, the family should explain the situation to his doctor as thoroughly as possible and then abide by the doctor's suggestions as to how to approach the patient. Such instances happen in our Clinic with great regularity, and usually, if the patient is approached in a knowledgeable man-ner, the situation is resolved without great difficulty.

Children

Patients with children present unique problems. When it is necessary to bring a young mother into the Sanctuary as an inpatient, we must consider what to do with her children. Occasionally an infant is brought into the Clinic with the mother. Most school-age children are left at home, under the care of the father, grandmother or friends. While I do not believe in separating mother and child, in certain severe forms of CFS there is no alternative.

Depending on the age of the child, he should be taught as completely as possible the nature of his mother's problem. No fanciful stories should be made up, as these can cause severe problems at a later date. Almost any child from the age of four up can be told what is "wrong with Mommy." The condition can be explained in language that a child can at least accept, even though he cannot fully understand. If there is real difficulty toward this end, the doctor should speak with the child. In my practice, I do this frequently, and often I am able to enlist better cooperation from the children than I can from many of the adults. Children should know that the CFS patient needs understanding and encouragement from them as much as from any other family member. A child's words of encouragement can be of great help to a loving mother.

While most of the foregoing discussion applies particularly to severe CFS cases who come as inpatients, the same information is helpful for those who remain as outpatients. In some ways the aid and cooperation of friends and family is even more important to outpatients, because while the inpatient's family contact is only intermittent, the outpatient's family contact is constant and, if poor in support and encouragement, the stress produced can be severe and unremitting.

Laws of Vibration

In Chapter Three we alluded to the vibratory states that surround the CFS patient. Perhaps a word of explanation would help to understand more fully what is meant by "vibratory states." By its atomic nature, all life puts out certain emanations which we know as vibrations. These have various effects and purposes, most of which it is not necessary to discuss here. The human being is no exception to this rule. In fact, since the human body is a heat-producing structure with electromagnetic and chemical reactions going on by the billions every second, it produces a strong vibratory or electro-magnetic field about itself. This field is affected by the basic electromagnetic and chemical structure of the body, by foods we eat, by the character of our elimination, by the thoughts we think, by the emotions which are prevalent within us, and even by our future aspirations as they affect the physical, mental and emotional components of our bodies. We all know people we instantly like and feel comfortable with; we also know people who leave us cold or unsettled and whom we would just as soon not see again. In these instances, we are affected by the aggregate of their vibratory forces in relationship to our own. In the first instance, the individual's vibratory forces are such that they reinforce and strengthen our own, while in the second, exactly the opposite effect is produced. This response is particularly strong in those with CFS. If they are around persons who are understanding and supportive, they can be swept along on this support, and great improvement can be brought about. If there are persons about the patient whose vibratory elements are antipathetic, the results produced are detrimental, and the patient's progress can be impeded by these forces of unsympathetic vibrations. It is not even neces-sary for those around the patient to communicate disap-proval. The mere presence of a person who is not understand-ing, harmonious and encouraging can be, and usually is, injurious to the patient's progress.

Summary

In a few words, the best routes for family and friends to take to help the CFS patient are: First, and by far the greatest, be understanding. The more these key people understand the patient's condition, the more they can say and do the correct thing at the proper time. Second, this knowledge must be put to good use in the form of the encouragement they give the patient along the way of his long and arduous road to recovery. He needs encouragement in the same way that a woman in love wants to hear the words, "I love you." A woman can never be told "I love you" too often, nor can the CFS patient be given too much encouragement. Even if you have told the patient an hour before that he is going to be all right, tell him again because it is on these words that he must live during an important part of his therapy program. Finally, friends should help the CFS patient keep his eye on his goal; do not let him wander into different pathways. It is easy for him to wander, because his journey is often long, and as on all long journeys, he begins to wonder if he has taken the right road. Let the patient know that he is on the right road and that he must continue on it to the end. If there is any doubt as to any part of his treatment, friends and family should have him speak to his doctor, or do so themselves. Unless the physician has the patient's confidence and the family's cooperation and assistance, recovery from CFS is almost impossible. The doctor can and must do a great deal in the treatment of these patients; but, he is capable of accomplishing this full task only with the help of the patient's friends and/or relatives, and most importantly, with the cooperation and efforts of the patient himself. Friends and relatives form an important—even a vital—part of recovery. If they do their task—as the doctor does his—and the patient cooperates, there may be complete assurance that the patient will be returned to a vital, productive existence.

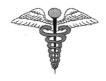

Chapter Five

The Hans Selye Chart and the Adrenal Stress Index

 NE of the most frustrating factors of Chronic Fatigue Syndrome (CFS) is that it seemingly does not correspond to any form of medical precedents or patterns. We do not deny that this is true, but personally feel that the fault is not so much in the condition as it is in the physicians who are not able to adapt to this unique type of problem. Once the physician is able to forget his usual concepts of treatment and cure and examine the physiology of the patient with an open mind and an inquiring heart, the fog and mist enshrouding CFS dissipate, and the pure solar rays of reason and logic will illuminate what was once obscure and opaque.

In Chapter Two, "History of the Disease," we described the many men of good heart and keen scientific mind who have addressed this problem with such reason and logic in past years. Unfortunately, very few physicians are aware of the work of these great pioneers. While it is not for us to judge, the lack of substantial financial gain to be made from this field of medicine may well have played an important part in this neglect. CFS is not a medical money-maker. To treat it properly takes a great deal of the doctor's time and energy. There are no simple get- rich-quick schemes with CFS as there are in conditions that have the potential of an expensive surgery. I have little doubt that if someone discovered an expensive brain operation that supposedly could be used to benefit the

CFS patient, you would see physicians' interest in this condition soar.

The truth is that there will never be such an operation. Nor will there be a drug that cures CFS. It just is not that kind of condition. It is simply the consequence of two factors, as explained in Chapter Three, "The Nature of the Patient": the inherited nature of the patient and the degree of unremitting stress under which he exists or existed. Not too much can be done about a patient's heredity, but most certainly the physician has an obligation to help the patient master his stresses.

In this chapter we will attempt to correlate the work of Dr. Hans Selye with the more modern Adrenal Stress Index (ASI) test. Once the patient and doctor have a working understanding of these two essential aids to a real cure of CFS, they will be able to move forward with a real healing protocol, instead of just treating symptoms with drugs or other stimulating substances that only make the condition worse in the long run.

In our experience, the entire secret of successfully treating CFS depends on a full understanding by both patient and physician of the following chart, "The Biologic Reaction to Stress," created by Dr. Hans Selye. This classic chart outlines the various stages of CFS dramatically, thus giving evidence to our contention that CFS is nothing more or less than the body's biological reaction to long-term unremitting stress.

As you can see from the Selye chart, it matters little what sort of stress the individual is encountering or has encountered; the end result is always the same. The body has a certain reaction to such unremitting stress, and the mechanism is always the same, since the body cannot tell one stress from another. It matters little to the body if your stress is emotional, mental or physical. It only measures amount, not the distinct type. However, the patient and the doctor do need to address the type of stress in order to help reduce it for the needed cure.

Many CFS patients report to us that their condition started with an infection of some sort, and they wonder if some unknown virus is not the real cause of CFS. I don't think so. Many investigators have attempted to discover the "bug" that

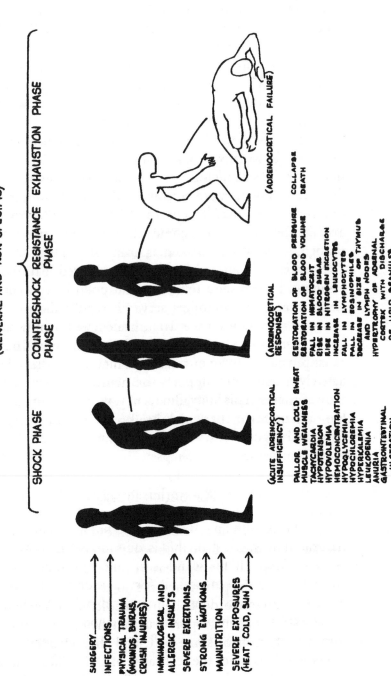

THE BIOLOGIC REACTION TO STRESS

STRESSORS

ALARM REACTION (SELYE)
(GENERAL AND NON-SPECIFIC)

SHOCK PHASE | COUNTERSHOCK PHASE | RESISTANCE PHASE | EXHAUSTION PHASE

SURGERY
INFECTIONS
PHYSICAL TRAUMA (WOUNDS, BURNS, CRUSH INJURIES)
IMMUNOLOGICAL AND ALLERGIC INSULTS
SEVERE EXERTIONS
STRONG EMOTIONS
MALNUTRITION
SEVERE EXPOSURES (HEAT, COLD, SUN)

(ACUTE ADRENOCORTICAL INSUFFICIENCY)

PALLOR AND COLD SWEAT
MUSCLE WEAKNESS
TACHYCARDIA
HYPOTENSION
HYPOVOLEMIA
HEMOCONCENTRATION
HYPOGLYCEMIA
HYPOCHLOREMIA
HYPERKALEMIA
LEUKOPENIA
ANURIA
GASTROINTESTINAL ULCERATION

(ADRENOCORTICAL RESPONSE)

RESTORATION OF BLOOD PRESSURE
RESTORATION OF BLOOD VOLUME
FALL IN HEMATOCRIT
RISE IN BLOOD SUGAR
RISE IN NITROGEN EXCRETION
INCREASE IN LEUKOCYTES
FALL IN LYMPHOCYTES
FALL IN EOSINOPHILES
DECREASE IN SIZE OF THYMUS AND LYMPH NODES
HYPERTROPHY OF ADRENAL CORTEX WITH DISCHARGE OF LIPID GRANULES

(ADRENOCORTICAL FAILURE)

COLLAPSE
DEATH

is the "real" cause of CFS, but so far none of them has been successful. At one time, the Epstein-Barr virus was thought by some to be the cause of this condition; however, as more rational minds looked at this matter they discovered that the Epstein-Barr virus is only, like many others, an opportunistic invader that is able to become a problem in the body when the immune system is compromised by CFS.

Personally, I would be very pleased if someone could discover a bug that we could eliminate to cure CFS. It would make my life so much easier. I could then really retire and devote my time to more personal endeavors. However, once one understands the Selye chart and listens to the history of the average CFS patient, it becomes clear that such an outcome, though devoutly to be wished, is simply not in the cards. The CFS patient has abused his body, or allowed it to become assaulted by exposure to toxins and pollution, to such an extent that it can no longer serve his regular daily requirements. It's just that simple. To be healed, we not only have to stop the past abuse (mental, physical and emotional), but also must pursue a course of treatment that, both passively and actively, builds and supports the neurohormonal and immune systems of his body. But let us now take a more detailed look at the Selye chart and "walk" an individual through Chronic Fatigue from a normal adrenal system to the development of adrenocortical collapse:

The Shock Phase

We begin with an individual who has a certain degree of natural vitality. Most of this is due to the integrity of the adrenal gland. If this gland is strong, the individual may endure a great deal of stress before developing the effects of Selye's first or Shock Phase. If an individual is not so lucky, or the stresses are so strong that despite a good constitution his body enters Dr. Selye's Shock Phase, these changes take place in the body:

Pallor and cold sweat. (We still see signs of this in CFS patients who are well past the Shock Phase. One of the things we do when we take our standard postural blood pressures is to feel the palms of the patient. If they are moist, we know the patient is still experiencing some effects of this Shock Phase.)

Muscle Weakness. This is due to the adrenal gland directing its vitality from the functioning of the body to its attempt to reestablish homeostasis, that is, body equilibrium.

Tachycardia. The heart speeds up in an effort to bring more blood to the vital organs to overcome the stress.

Hypotension. The blood pressure drops, as the adrenal is not able to maintain the normal pressure. This is especially evident in the drop in blood pressure the patient experiences when he suddenly stands up after having been reclining (the orthostatic blood pressure test).

Hypovolemia. There is lowering of the blood volume.

Hemoconcentration. Due to the lower blood volume there is a concentration of the red and white blood cells.

Hypoglycemia. The blood sugar goes down as the body attempts to use more of it to boost the organs in a state of shock.

Hypochloremia. The chlorine concentration in the blood is reduced. This may also lower the ability of the body to make sufficient hydrochloric acid and thus impede digestion. Poor digestion is a common problem with the CFS patient.

Hyperkalemia. The potassium content of the blood is raised.

Leukopenia. There is a lowering of the white blood cell count.

Anuria. The amount of urine is reduced.

Gastrointestinal Ulceration. The immune system is stressed and allows the integrity of the intestinal mucosa to become susceptible to ulceration.

These reactions are most pronounced in the acute stage of adrenocortical insufficiency, but this is a state we see rarely in our Clinic. Usually this stage of adrenal insufficiency sneaks up on the individual who develops CFS. The most common symptoms experienced are spells of fatigue and muscle weakness that frequently come and go.

When we take the history of a CFS patient he usually confesses to us that he has had times in the past when he had some of these symptoms but disregarded them and just "pushed" a little harder to get his work done. If he sought medical help, the a physician usually gave him something to "pep him up" or told him to exercise more to build up his muscle tone. Of course, the final result of all these efforts was to force his body into mobilizing the Hypothalamic–Pituitary Axis to overstimulate the adrenal gland and, thus, move the individual forward (as far as the Selye chart is concerned) into the Countershock and Resistance Phases.

The Countershock and Resistance Phases

When we look at the Selye chart, it is confusing at first to see that the figure in the Countershock Phase is looking better than the figure in the previous phase, that the figure in the Resistance Phase appears the same as the normal figure, and that the next stage after the good-looking Resistance Phase is severe exhaustion and complete adrenal collapse. Since most of the patients who come to us are in the Countershock Phase or the Resistance Phase, it is important that we clarify the nature of these two phases as much as possible.

The individual who properly treats the first or Shock Phase of Dr. Selye will not go on to develop "chronic" CFS. It is only when this early stage is ignored or mistreated that the person advances into the later stages. Unfortunately, the dedicated, responsible individual (the one most likely to develop CFS) is also the person who is inclined to continue to push his body until it is forced to take the countershock measures described by Dr. Selye. Once the body is forced into the Countershock Phase, the individual enters an advanced stage of CFS and is on his way to a great deal of suffering and frustration.

If we compare these phases with what happens to an individual's personal finances, it might make the situation a little clearer. The Shock Phase of the Selye chart may be compared to a person who has suddenly lost his job (a true shock to be sure). His income is greatly reduced, and if he is wise he will learn to live within his new lower funds until he can find new employment. Let us say, however, that he does not want to live within his new means and begins to use his bank account to sustain him in the life-style he was used to before he lost his job. This use of his savings would allow him to keep the same life-style as before, and his friends would notice no change in him. The only trouble with this scenario is that eventually his bank account will run out, and then he is in real trouble.

Even if he should be able to find a job before his bank account is fully exhausted, he still has depleted it severely and must either become very frugal in the future so he can rebuild this emergency account or take the chance of living with a diminished bank account.

So is it with the CFS patient. The first stages of the Shock Phase are like losing one's job. The body's vitality (adrenal integrity) has been compromised by some combination of stresses, and the patient needs to reduce his level of activity (adjust his life-style) until he is able to renew the adrenal's integrity (find a new job). If this is not done, that is, if he forces his body to go to its emergency stores of energy, they will gradually be depleted. Unless something is not done quickly to correct this situation, he will move to the later phases of the Selye chart. Thus we see that while the Countershock and Resistance Phases may look good on the chart (as may the man living on his life savings), they are a dangerous place to live and will create a wide variety of undesirable symptoms in the patient.

In the Countershock and Resistance Phases we find the following responses by the body:

Restoration of the Blood Pressure. What we often find in our patients in this stage is that the postural blood pressure (blood pressure taken lying down and then standing) will show an accentuated rise when the patient stands up. In a severe case, the longer the patient stands, the higher the pressure will go. The adrenal mechanism has become so over-sensitized that even the slightest stimulus will set it off, giving these patients their own special form of hell.

Restoration of Blood Volume. This accompanies the rise in blood pressure.

Fall in Hematocrit. With the greater blood volume the red blood cells are now more diluted, and so their concentration is reduced.

Rise in Blood Sugar. This rise helps to overcome the symptoms of hypoglycemia that are a part of the original Shock Phase. However, in our experience this is only tempo-rary, and some patients in these phases continue to have low blood sugar problems as the condition advances.

Rise in Nitrogen Excretion. Patients are often agitated by the elevated cortisol levels present in these phases, and this will make it difficult to gain weight. The body may also lose muscle mass due to nitrogen excretion (nitrogen is an essential com-ponent of protein).

Increase in Leukocytes. Fall in Lymphocytes. Fall in Eosinophils. These changes are due to the emergency mode the body has had to assume. It is prepared to fight an acute infection by the relatively increased neutrophils (the white blood cells that fight acute infections best). However, since the immune system is depressed by the elevated cortisol levels, we have a situation in which we have a big army of foot soldiers but very few arms and ammunition for them to fight with.

Decrease in the Size of Thymus and Lymph Nodes. It is the thymus and lymph nodes that must give the body the backup support for any infective emergencies. As described above, the elevated cortisols triggered by these phases depress the immune response (the thymus and lymph nodes).

Hypertrophy of Adrenal Cortex with Discharge of Lipid Granules. In an effort to meet the needs of the body's stress, the adrenal cortex enlarges, but this is much like the thyroid enlargement in goiter. This enlargement of the adrenal cortex is a near-useless attempt to provide the body with something that it can no longer manage—normal adrenal activity.

Most patients who come to our Clinic are in the Counter-shock or Resistance Phase of CFS. Occasionally a patient will come to us in the second Exhaustion Phase, but thank goodness these are few and far between. Once in a while we will see a patient in the first or Shock Phase, but usually these individuals are first seen by a local practitioner, either traditional or alternative. The usual treatment given these "beginning" CFS patients is frequently such that they finally end up in the later stages of this condition; that is when they come to see us.

Synopsis of the Adrenal Stress Progression

As you can see from the Selye chart, a typical CFS patient has usually been exposed to a variety of stresses that he is not able to resolve until finally the body is not able to adapt and he enters the Shock, or first exhaustion, Phase. This is identical to the weakness one experiences after a serious infection (like a strong case of influenza) or other severe stress on the system like an automobile accident or some other trauma. If the individual will take the time to rest until the stressed organs (particularly the adrenal glands) have an opportunity to regenerate from the stressful situation, his glandular system will return to normal and not advance to the Countershock and Resistance Phases of CFS. Unfortunately, what usually happens is that the CFS-prone individual is so conscientious that he forces himself to return to his regular daily tasks before the stressed glands have a chance to return to normal.

If this lack of strength is small, the patient will notice little change in his ability to function but his glandular and nervous system have been compromised. The next time this happens, the gland system becomes a little more compromised since it was weaker to start with than in the first episode. Since the nature of the CFS-susceptible individual is to keep going under all circumstances, this scenario is repeated time and again until some stress so overwhelms the gland system that it is not able to regenerate as before and the individual begins to experience the full-blown symptoms of CFS.

As discussed in an earlier chapter, the amount of stress needed to bring on this phase where the glands cannot create the effect of normalcy varies greatly from individual to individual. In persons with serious hereditary weakness of the adrenals it may take only one or two episodes before CFS rears its ugly head. In others it may take many, and as discussed before, in some whose inherited gland system is very strong it may never occur.

Once the gland system has reached the point at which it cannot readily regenerate itself, it must be helped by outside efforts by both the patient and a physician knowledgeable in treating this condition. Too often instead of real help the new CFS patient is given only a "Band-aid" and the condition gradually advances into the later phases. We can see this progression in the three ASI tests of actual CFS patients that follow.

Typical ASI Tests

As you can see in the first ASI test (pp. 100-101), all the cortisol levels are above normal, but the DHEA levels are at a borderline low. This is the ASI of the typical Countershock and Resistance Phase patient. This is the test of a career woman who has had to push her body to keep up with the rigors of her job. Her Hypothalamic–Pituitary Axis has become so sensitive that it is almost constantly stimulating the adrenals to pour forth more and more hormones to meet her daily needs. In doing so, it has depleted her stores of hormone precursors (DHEAs) to a dangerous level. Unless she is properly treated and the Hypothalamic–Pituitary Axis sensitivity reduced, she will soon run out of raw material for her hormones and then her condition will degenerate into the second Exhaustion Phase. Her below-normal Salivary Secretory IgA shows the inhibition of her immune system by the elevated cortisol levels.

The symptoms of a patient in her stage of CFS are a mixture of fatigue and anxiety. Sometimes both will manifest at the same time (something that only another CFS patient can fully appreciate or comprehend), but usually these two symtoms will alternate.

In the second ASI test (pp. 102-103), we find a patient who is beginning to pass from the Resistance Phase into the second Exhaustion Phase. The DHEA levels have dropped below normal, and therefore, since the adrenal gland does not have the raw material it needs to respond to the stimulus of the Hypothalamic–Pituitary Axis,[1] the cortisol levels are beginning to descend. In this patient, the anxiety has begun to lessen with the descent of the cortisol levels, but as one might expect, the exhaustion is becoming more pervasive and unbearable. The cortisol levels may look normal to a physician who is not familiar with the idiosyncrasies of CFS, but there are two factors that let us know this patient's true situation—the low DHEA and IgA levels, both lower than those in the first patient's test. This latter reading (IgA) assures us that this patient has had high cortisol levels in the past which depressed

---

[1] The Hypothalamic–Pituitary Axis is that mechanism in the body that regulates the activity of the adrenal gland. It is the mechanism that stimulates the adrenal to pour out the needed hormones for fight or flight. It is so designed that it normally becomes active only when an emergency need for extra hormones exists. Once this emergency is over, this mechanism will cease stimulating the adrenal, thus giving this gland a chance to rebuild the hormones expended during the emergency. In the Counter-shock and Resistance Phases of Chronic Fatigue Syndrome the Hypothalamic–Pituitary Axis often will attempt to constantly stimulate the adrenal to activity to make up for the weakness of this gland. By doing so, it is only whipping a tired horse and steadily depleting the body's stores of DHEAs, the precursors of the adrenal and other hormones of the body. In order to correct this abnormal situation, it is necessary to "convince" this Hypothalamic–Pituitary Axis mechanism that there is no emergency so that it will cease its near-constant stimulation of the adrenal gland. This calming down of the Hypothalamic–Pituitary Axis is accomplished by the use of a nutritional remedy containing a phosphorylated serine and by the various passive therapies used at our Clinic. Unless this reduction in activity of the Hypothalamic–Pituitary Axis is accomplished, patients in the Counter-shock and Resistance Phases of Chronic Fatigue Syndrome will not return to the normal functioning they desire. (See Chapter Nine for details.)

Diagnos-Techs, Inc.
Clinical & Research Laboratory
PO BOX 58948, Seattle, WA 98138-1948
Tel: (425) 251-0596

CLIA License # 50D0630141

Date Received: 03/20/98
Collection Date: 03/16/98

Report Date: 04/20/98

(c) 1987-1998 by Diagnos-Techs, Inc.
All Rights Reserved.

Accession: 98-06733

Results for:

GERALD POESNECKER ND
HEALING RESEARCH CENTER
5916 CLYMER RD
QUAKERTOWN, PA 18951

FAX: 1(215)536-9099

Test	Description	Result		Ref Values	
ASI	ADRENAL STRESS INDEX				KEY FOR DHEA-CORTISOL CORRELATION
TAP	TEMPORAL ADRENAL PROFILE				1. Stress adapted "hyper" response: minimal changes.
	Free Cortisol Values: (nM - Nano Molar)				2. Stress adapted with a divergence in response to ACTH.
	7:00 - 8:00 AM	25	Borderline	13 - 23	3. Maladaptation Phase I.
	11:00 - 12:00 PM	21	Elevated	5 - 10	4. Maladaptation Phase II.
	4:00 - 5:00 PM	12	Elevated	3 - 8	5. Adrenal fatigue, non-adapted.
	11:00 - 11:59 PM	8	Elevated	1 - 3	6. Inappropriate DHEAS with non ACTH dependent stimulation.
	Cortisol Time Integral: 66			23 - 42	7. Adrenal failure.
DHEA & DHEA(S)		3	Borderline	3 - 10 ng/ml (Adult)	

===
Low DHEA is a normal finding in children below age 14 and DHEA augmentation is NOT APPLICABLE
===

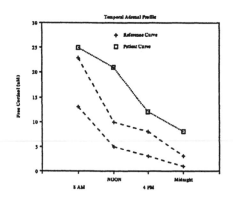

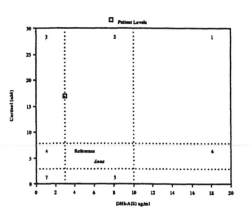

Diagnos-Techs, Inc.

Clinical & Research Laboratory
PO BOX 58948, Seattle, WA 98138-1948
Tel: (425) 251-0596

CLIA License # 50D0630141

Date Received: 03/20/98

Collection Date: 03/16/98

Report Date: 04/20/98

Results continued for:

Accession: 98-06733

Test	Description	Result	Ref Values

MUCOSAL BARRIER SCREEN

Test	Description	Result	Ref Values
MB2S	Salivary Secretory IgA	13.00	Normal: 25-60 mg/dl Borderline: 20 - 25 Depressed: < 20 Elevated: > 60
MB5S	ANTI-GLIADIN SIgA	1	Positive: > 15 U/ml Borderline: 13 - 15 U/ml Negative: < 13 U/ml

Gliadin Antibodies SIgA (AGA) Interpretation:

Gliadins are polypeptides found in wheat, rye, oat, barley, and other grain glutens. Specific toxic gliadins are responsible for the insulting effect of grains to the intestinal mucosa in susceptible individuals.

Presentation of Gliadin sensitivity in Overt celiac disease includes: Multiple vitamin and mineral deficiencies, steatorrhea, general weakness, diarrhea, and bone pain.

Subclinical and undetected Gliadin sensitivity may show unobvious symptoms and findings including: Mild enteritis, occasional loose stools, fat intolerance, marginal vitamin and mineral status, fatigue, or accelerated osteoporosis.

Differential Diagnosis: Positive AGA titer. AGA Negative or significantly reduced following 2-3 months of treatment. Treatment depends on severity. For example, mild to moderate subclinical cases require rotation or reduction in gluten intake. Overt Celiac disease requires avoidance of gluten.

Positive AGA or elevated AGA antibodies may not necessarily imply a celiac disease state, but a subclinical mucotoxic reaction. Healthy Adults and Children may show positive antibodies to Gliadin. Scan. J. Gastroenterol. 29:248(1994). Interpret results with discretion.

REMARKS

Please rule out the presence of hormone mediated pathologies before hormone augmentation or replacement therapies are initiated.

COURTESY INTERPRETATIONS of tests and Technical Support are available upon request, to Physicians Only.

Diagnos-Techs, Inc.

Clinical & Research Laboratory
PO BOX 58948, Seattle, WA 98138-1948
Tel: (425) 251-0596

CLIA License # 50D0630141

Date Received: 06/17/98

Collection Date: 06/14/98

Report Date: 06/20/98

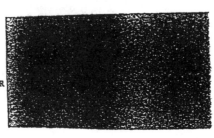

Accession: 98-14480

GERALD POESNECKER ND
HEALING RESEARCH CENTER
5916 CLYMER RD
QUAKERTOWN, PA 18951

FAX: 1(215)536-9099

Test	Description	Result	Ref Values
ASI	ADRENAL STRESS INDEX		
TAP	TEMPORAL ADRENAL PROFILE		

KEY FOR DHEA-CORTISOL CORRELATION

1. Stress adapted "hyper" response: minimal changes.

Free Cortisol Values: (nM - Nano Molar)

2. Stress adapted with a divergence in response to ACTH.

Time	Result	Status	Ref
7:00 - 8:00 AM	23	Normal	13 - 23
11:00 - 12:00 PM	10	Borderline	5 - 10
4:00 - 5:00 PM	6	Normal	3 - 8
11:00 - 11:59 PM	2	Normal	1 - 3
Cortisol Time Integral: 41			23 - 42

3. Maladaptation Phase I.

4. Maladaptation Phase II.

5. Adrenal fatigue, non-adapted.

6. Inappropriate DHEAS with non ACTH dependent stimulation.

7. Adrenal failure.

DHEA & DHEA(S)　　2　　Depressed　3 - 10 ng/ml (Adult)

==
Low DHEA is a normal finding in children below age 14 and DHEA augmentation is NOT APPLICABLE
==

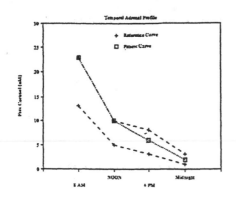

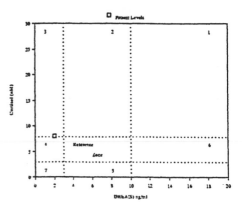

Diagnos-Techs, Inc.

Clinical & Research Laboratory
PO BOX 58948. Seattle. WA 98138-1948
Tel: (425) 251-0596

CLIA License # 50D0630141

Date Received: 06/17/98
Collection Date: 06/14/98

Report Date: 06/20/98

(c) 1987-1998 by Diagnos-Techs. Inc.
All Rights Reserved.

Test	Description	Result	Ref Values
MUCOSAL BARRIER SCREEN			
MB2S	Salivary Secretory IgA	8.00	Normal: 25-60 mg/dl Borderline: 20 - 25 Depressed: < 20 Elevated: > 60
MB5S	ANTI-GLIADIN SIgA	1	Positive: > 15 U/ml Borderline: 13 - 15 U/ml Negative: < 13 U/ml

Gliadin Antibodies SIgA (AGA) Interpretation:

Gliadins are polypeptides found in wheat, rye, oat, barley, and other grain glutens. Specific toxic gliadins are responsible for the insulting effect of grains to the intestinal mucosa in susceptible individuals.

Presentation of Gliadin sensitivity in Overt celiac disease includes: Multiple vitamin and mineral deficiencies, steatorrhea, general weakness, diarrhea, and bone pain.

Subclinical and undetected Gliadin sensitivity may show unobvious symptoms and findings including: Mild enteritis, occasional loose stools, fat intolerance, marginal vitamin and mineral status, fatigue, or accelerated osteoporosis.

Differential Diagnosis: Positive AGA titer. AGA Negative or significantly reduced following 2-3 months of treatment. Treatment depends on severity. For example, mild to moderate subclinical cases require rotation or reduction in gluten intake. Overt Celiac disease requires avoidance of gluten.

Positive AGA or elevated AGA antibodies may not necessarily imply a celiac disease state, but a subclinical mucotoxic reaction. Healthy Adults and Children may show positive antibodies to Gliadin. Scan. J. Gastroenterol. 29:248(1994). Interpret results with discretion.

REMARKS

Please rule out the presence of hormone mediated pathologies before hormone augmentation or replacement therapies are initiated.

COURTESY INTERPRETATIONS of tests and Technical Support are available upon request, to Physicians Only.

Diagnos-Techs, Inc.

Clinical & Research Laboratory
PO BOX 58948, Seattle, WA 98138-1948
Tel: (425) 251-0596

CLIA License # 50D0630141

Date Received: 03/04/98
Collection Date: 03/01/98

Report Date: 03/06/98

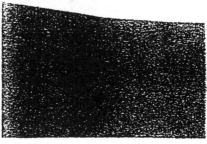

Accession: 98-05189

GERALD POESNECKER ND
HEALING RESEARCH CENTER
5916 CLYMER RD
QUAKERTOWN, PA 18951

FAX: 1(215)536-9099

Test	Description	Result	Ref Values
ASI	ADRENAL STRESS INDEX		KEY FOR DHEA-CORTISOL CORRELATION

TAP   TEMPORAL ADRENAL PROFILE

1. Stress adapted "hyper" response; minimal changes.

Free Cortisol Values: (nM - Nano Molar)

2. Stress adapted with a divergence in response to ACTH.

7:00 - 8:00 AM	2	Depressed	13 - 23	3. Maladaptation Phase I.
11:00 - 12:00 PM	3	Depressed	5 - 10	4. Maladaptation Phase II.
4:00 - 5:00 PM	2	Depressed	3 - 8	5. Adrenal fatigue, non-adapted.
11:00 - 11:59 PM	2	Normal	1 - 3	6. Inappropriate DHEAS with non ACTH dependent stimulation.
Cortisol Time Integral: 9			23 - 42	7. Adrenal failure.

DHEA & DHEA(S)   1   Depressed   3 - 10 ng/ml (Adult)

===
Low DHEA is a normal finding in children below age 14 and DHEA augmentation is NOT APPLICABLE
===

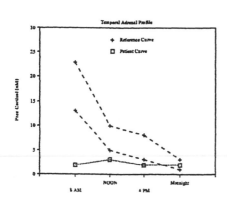

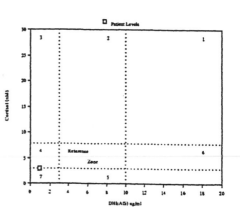

Diagnos-Techs, Inc.

Date Received: 03/04/98

Collection Date: 03/01/98

Clinical & Research Laboratory
PO BOX 58948, Seattle, WA 98138-1948
Tel: (425) 251-0596

Report Date: 03/06/98

CLIA License # 50D0630141

(c) 1987-1998 by Diagnos-Techs, Inc.
All Rights Reserved.

Results continued for:

Accession: 97-15785

Test	Description	Result	Ref Values

MUCOSAL BARRIER SCREEN

MB2S	Salivary Secretory IgA	4.00	Normal: 25-60 mg/dl
			Borderline: 20 - 25
			Depressed: < 20
			Elevated: > 60

MB5S	ANTI-GLIADIN SIgA	4	Positive: > 15 U/ml
			Borderline: 13 - 15 U/ml
			Negative: < 13 U/ml

Gliadin Antibodies SIgA (AGA) Interpretation:

Gliadins are polypeptides found in wheat, rye, oat, barley, and other grain glutens. Specific toxic gliadins are responsible for the insulting effect of grains to the intestinal mucosa in susceptible individuals.

Presentation of Gliadin sensitivity in Overt celiac disease includes: Multiple vitamin and mineral deficiencies, steatorrhea, general weakness, diarrhea, and bone pain.

Subclinical and undetected Gliadin sensitivity may show unobvious symptoms and findings including: Mild enteritis, occasional loose stools, fat intolerance, marginal vitamin and mineral status, fatigue, or accelerated osteoporosis.

Differential Diagnosis: Positive AGA titer. AGA Negative or significantly reduced following 2-3 months of treatment. Treatment depends on severity. For example, mild to moderate subclinical cases require rotation or reduction in gluten intake. Overt Celiac disease requires avoidance of gluten.

Positive AGA or elevated AGA antibodies may not necessarily imply a celiac disease state, but a subclinical mucotoxic reaction. Healthy Adults and Children may show positive antibodies to Gliadin. Scan. J. Gastroenterol. 29:248(1994). Interpret results with discretion.

REMARKS

Please rule out the presence of hormone mediated pathologies before hormone augmentation or replacement therapies are initiated.

COURTESY INTERPRETATIONS of tests and Technical Support are available upon request, to Physicians Only.

her immune system, even though such elevated cortisol is not now in evidence.

This patient needs a great deal of help. She is an excellent patient to come into our Sanctuary for treatment, since she needs to have her stresses reduced to a minimum and her treatment extended to the maximum—something that is very difficult to do in most home environments.

In the third pictured ASI chart, we find an individual in a full-blown second Exhaustion Phase.[2] As you can see from the very low cortisol levels, there is very little, if any, influence that the Hypothalamic–Pituitary Axis is exerting on the adrenal gland. This fact is shown by the uniformly low cortisol levels throughout the day. When we examine the DHEA levels in this patient, we can see the cause for the ineffectiveness of the

---

[2] What Dr. Selye calls the Shock Phase we like to call the first Exhaustion Phase since this describes the symptoms of Chronic Fatigue Syndrome patients better during this stage of their condition. There definitely is exhaustion during this stage of the condition, but this exhaustion will abate under one of two scenarios. In the first scenario, if the patient gives his glandular system a full chance to regenerate following the stresses that brought on this first phase of adrenal exhaustion, his gland will return to normal and he will move from right to left on the Selye chart and his exhaustion will eventually leave. In the second scenario, the patient does not give his glandular system a chance to regenerate, but rather keeps pushing it until, in an effort to establish some sort of equilibrium, the body is forced into the Countershock Phase. In this phase, as shown by the Selye chart, his exhaustion begins to be replaced by a strange form of anxiety plus weakness known only to those Chronic Fatigue Syndrome patients who experience it. They are weak and exhausted, but have great difficulty in resting or sleeping due to the various body changes created to produce the Countershock Phase.

In the second Exhaustion Phase we have a different situation entirely from that in the first one. Before this phase, the body has attempted to support the needs of the individual by using its emergency stores of energy. The individual passes into this second Exhaustion Phase only when these stores are nearly depleted. There simply is not enough raw material left to produce the effects of the Countershock or Resistance Phases any longer. The cortisol levels drop, and a state of severe exhaustion ensues that cannot, unlike the first stage exhaustion, be relieved by the body's motivation of emergency stores of vitality. There are none left to activate.

Hypothalamic–Pituitary Axis—there are not enough DHEAs available to produce the needed hormones even with the full stimulation of the Hypothalamic–Pituitary Axis.

Also note that even with the complete lack of elevated cortisol inhibition, the IgA levels are even lower than the other two ASI tests. In our experience, once the high cortisol levels of the Countershock and Resistance Phases have depressed the immune system, it will not rise again unless the patient's adrenals are regenerated by a move from the right to the left on the Selye chart.

Out of respect for the great Dr. Hans Selye, we have kept his chart exactly as it was handed down to us. While it is nearly perfect for our use in CFS, that was not its original purpose. Dr. Selye was attempting to illustrate what would happen to the body as it went through various changes in response to stress. His main objective was to show how the body responds to the acute forms of severe stress. He viewed, as the final outcome of this process, complete adrenalcortical failure—leading finally to death. While this may happen in times of war and other dramatic traumas, this does not occur in the CFS patient. His condition is chronic rather than acute, and the events taking place according to Dr. Selye's chart progress so slowly that the body has time to adapt. Thus the end game for the Chronic Fatigue patient is not death, but rather a near vegetative, exhausted existence. In my experience treating CFS I have never seen a patient die of this condition. However, I have seen many so weak and exhausted that they were not able to leave their bed and must be waited upon hand and foot. This, not death, is the final outcome of an untreated or ineffectively treated case of CFS.

Conclusion

Within this chapter is found the real secret of treating CFS. Every person with this condition resides somewhere on the chart of Dr. Selye. If they do not, they don't have CFS. All too many doctors are looking for the triggering mechanism that may have set off the initial symptom pattern. This is basically a useless endeavor, because this will be different with every person and is not the real cause of the condition. No matter what the triggering mechanism may be, the underlying effect on the patient's adrenal system is always the same. It is vital for the CFS patient to realize that it is not knowledge about the triggering event (that final stress that caused the CFS symptoms to manifest) that is important for his final recovery, but rather the degree of the underlying weakness of his adrenal glandular system and what methods and treatments are chosen to regenerate (not stimulate) this system to normal functioning once again.

In our work, we deem it essential to know exactly where the CFS patient is in relation to the Selye chart. While there are several laboratories that now test the saliva for DHEA and cortisol levels, we have found a specific laboratory whose results most closely agree with the clinical symptoms of our patients. This is the laboratory we use routinely for all our Chronic Fatigue patients. All the ASI tests in this book are from this source. We will not at this time attempt to treat a CFS patient without such an ASI test. To do so is like attempting to set a complicated fracture without a diagnostic x ray of the affected area.

If they expect to improve and return to normal, all CFS patients must work from the right to left on the Selye chart and cannot skip any of the Phases in their return to normal. If you are in the Resistance Phase you cannot expect to jump to the normal stage (the goal we all have in mind) in one fell swoop. From the Resistance Phase you must proceed back through the Countershock Phase and the first Exhaustion Phase (Selye's Shock Phase) before you will be able to return to normal. It is for this reason that CFS patients in the Countershock and Resistance Phases find that under proper treatment, their Hypothalamic–Pituitary Axis sensitivity is reduced and they have less of the anxiety that has plagued them so long. On the other hand, since they are not receiving the Hypothalamic–Pituitary Axis overstimulation, they will gradually become more relaxed, exhausted and seem to need more rest than before. As their overactive Hypothalamic–Pituitary Axis comes under further control with proper treatment, their abnormally high cortisol levels will begin to drop into the normal range and the "motor" that has been running wild inside of them for so long will finally cease entirely. However, they will now begin to feel the true state of weakness of their glandular system as it actually is and not as it was with the artificial stimulation of the overactive Hypothalamic–Pituitary Axis. They have now returned to the first Exhaustion Phase and are experiencing all the symptoms characteristic of that Phase. That is the bad news. The good news is that this is the last phase before the return to normal, so the patient should rejoice that the end of his long ordeal with CFS finally is near.

There is hope for every CFS patient. We have been treating this condition successfully for over four decades and can state, without fear of contradiction, that all patients, in all the different Selye phases, can be helped. Obviously, those in the earlier phases can expect good improvement faster than those in the later phases, but even here good improvement is to be expected in all patients who are willing to work with us toward that final recovery.

One last word of warning before we leave this chapter. By the time most patients come to us, they are in the latter phases of CFS. Their bodies and neurohormonal systems have been considerably altered by the processes described in the Selye chart. These various changes have been progressively taking place for several years by the time we begin treating most patients. We are not about to perform a quick miracle on these patients. It is going to take some time to return the many affected body systems to normal. It can be done, but it is not the work of a day, week or even a month. When I was the Director of the Clymer Health Clinic I had a statement I used when asked how long a condition would take to correct. I replied to the questioner, "I know you want a miracle and we are going to give you one, but it will be a *slow miracle.*"

Chapter Six

The Hypothalamic–Pituitary Axis

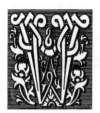 HILE we have mentioned the Hypothalamic–Pituitary Axis many times in our text, we find in actual practice that its importance cannot be overemphasized to the Chronic Fatigue Syndrome (CFS) patient during certain phases of his condition. It is this mechanism that produces some of the most agonizing effects of the CFS. If the patient is well-versed in the functioning of this Hypothalamic–Pituitary Axis, he can better understand his own symptom patterns and take measures to alleviate them. Before we get into the managing of this entity, however, we need to take a little time to define and explain just exactly what we are talking about.

The Hypothalamic–Pituitary Axis is the mechanism that stimulates the adrenal gland to greater activity when the need arises. It is not there for the usual day-to-day needs of the adrenal gland but for those emergencies that require a heroic effort on the part of this gland. For this reason it is called the "fight or flight" stimulant. If an emergency arises and the individual needs extra energy to fight or run, the hypothalamus and pituitary gland detect the need and send nerve and hormonal messengers to the adrenal gland to quickly increase its hormonal output to meet this sudden challenge. The adrenal does this by mobilizing various stores that it has been accumulating "for a rainy day." Once the emergency is over, the Hypothalamic–Pituitary Axis ceases its stimulation of the adrenal gland, and this gland is able to rest in order to replace its expended stores. It is for this reason that we are tired after such an effort and need rest and sleep to allow the adrenal gland to recuperate. This same effect can be seem after a bout of an acute infective disease. The adrenal must use its reserve stores to fight the infection, and therefore, once the infection is controlled by the body and the adrenal is able to rest, we feel very tired and weak for a few days. It is during this time that the adrenal has "withdrawn" to regenerate. If we give it time to do so, all will be well and it will be able to fully replace its expended stores, but if we attempt to force ourselves back to activity before all its stores are replaced, we set the stage for a possible later episode of CFS.

What happens with the Hypothalamic–Pituitary Axis in the CFS patient is either one of two things: Either his adrenal gland is so weak by nature (or by the treatment he had as a child) that the only way the body can stand up to the needs of his daily life is to force the Hypothalamic–Pituitary Axis to regularly overstimulate the weakened adrenal gland in a vain effort to help the patient maintain his chosen life-style. In my office I give patients the analogy of the whipping of an exhausted horse to get a little more effort out of him. In the second instance we have a patient who started out with a fairly normal adrenal gland but whose life-style involves such heavy unremitting stress[1] that eventually, here, too, the Hypothalamic–Pituitary Axis starts working overtime to meet the need. With each passing day the adrenal gland pours out more hormone than it is able to rebuild during its rare rest periods. It is like a person who takes a little out of his bank account to live on each day but replaces less than he removes. Eventually the day will come when the account is empty. This is when CFS rears its ugly head, and the patient cannot understand why this "suddenly" happens to him.

[1] By the term "unremitting stress" we are referring to those stresses that are of such an ongoing, all-pervasive nature that they do not allow the adrenal gland time to rest and regenerate between them as it would normally be able to do were these stresses more intermittent.

Invariably we find that there is a "straw that breaks the camel's back" in the average CFS patient's history. We are told of an infection or accident or a death of a loved one that he feels was the thing that caused the CFS. This is not true. This traumatic event is only the triggering factor in long line of unremitting stress. Had it not happened something else would have happened to act as a trigger in the not too distant future since the patient was obviously "ripe" for developing CFS.

Once CFS manifests, the Hypothalamic–Pituitary Axis takes on a new significance to both the patient and the physician. Unlike the adrenal gland this mechanism never seems to tire. It is especially active in the Countershock and Resistance Phases of CFS. In these stages it keeps up its efforts to stimulate the adrenal gland to fulfill the body's requirements. The mere fact that the adrenal gland is nearly exhausted does not seem to deter the Hypothalamic–Pituitary Axis from its efforts.

It is this combination of an exhausted adrenal gland and an overactive Hypothalamic–Pituitary Axis that produces a symptom pattern unique to CFS. That is the nearly simultaneous appearance of exhaustion and anxiety in the patient. While the patient is basically fatigued, he also feels as though he has a motor running inside him that just will not shut off. At night he is exhausted and needs sleep badly, but this motor will not allow him to really rest and sleep. What little sleep he gets does not satisfy, and he often wakes up in the morning more exhausted than when he went to bed.

Sometimes these two symptoms will alternate during the day. The patient may feel completely exhausted in the morning only to come alive in the evening, and then be so wound up that he can't sleep that night. In some CFS patients these two states will come and go from day to day with almost no seeming rationale. Still others may have several days of exhaustion to be followed by a day or two of anxiety and overstimulation. I had one patient who was on a one-day-on and one-day-off schedule that worked just like clockwork. One day she would be exhausted and the next overstimulated. The following day back to exhaustion. When we were able to break this pattern, she finally accepted that she was a CFS patient.

It is easy for some doctors to misdiagnose some of these patients as manic-depressive but they are not. The pattern of the true manic-depressive is much more prolonged than that of these CFS patients.

The mechanisms behind these multiple personalities are not that difficult to understand once we comprehend the interplay of the Hypothalamic–Pituitary Axis and the weakened adrenal gland. The exhausted times are when the adrenal gland is just too weak to respond to the stimulation of the Hypothalamic–Pituitary Axis. The patient is forced to rest at this time (they are too weak to do anything else), allowing the adrenal gland to regenerate a small amount. When this small amount of regeneration is sufficient to respond to the incessant stimulation of the Hypothalamic–Pituitary Axis, the patient will slip into the anxious mode and need to become active, or the "motor" within him will drive him to distraction. To the non-CFS patient the words and phrases used here will seem strange and enigmatic, but the CFS patient will know instantly to what I am referring.

To help these pitiful patients, we must attack their plight from two directions. We must first use special nutrient agents to modify the overreaction of the Hypothalamic–Pituitary Axis. Fortunately, we are able to do this with a product containing a phosphorylated mixture of L-Serine and Ethanolamine. This is not a drug, but a mixture of amino acid analogues that is able to convince the Hypothalamic–Pituitary Axis that the patient is not being constantly chased by a saber-toothed tiger. The phosphorylated mixture of L-Serine and Ethanolamine should be used only while being carefully monitored by a physician well versed in its use, because it is to be used only when the results of the ASI test show that it is needed, and even then only at those times when this test shows the Hypothalamic–Pituitary Axis overactivity. As mentioned before, there are no magic silver bullets to cure CFS. There are, however, some very useful tools, but like all tools, these are effective only in the hands of a practitioner who knows exactly how to use them to produce the desired effect.

The second and more difficult challenge to overcoming the adverse effects of this interplay between the weakened adrenal gland and an overactive Hypothalamic–Pituitary Axis is to train the patient not to do those things that will trigger the Hypothalamic–Pituitary Axis during our regenerative efforts. Once a patient in this vacillating phase of CFS starts to feel the exhaustion stage lift, even the slightest, he wants to be off and running, hoping against hope that maybe this time he is really cured and the exhaustion stage will not return. It always does, and his hopes are dashed on the rocks of reality once again. You would think that eventually he would learn, but it seems a very difficult lesson for the CFS patient to apply. However, no CFS patient is going to gain mastery over his condition until he is not only able to understand this lesson but is able to apply it on a daily basis. I make this statement from the monitoring of tens of thousands of patients for almost half a century.

But what is the patient to do? How would you have him react to the trials of this phase of CFS? First, he needs to understand as completely as possible the mechanisms going on in his body. This will give him a comprehension of what is actually happening when various symptoms manifest. This knowledge removes his fears of the unknown.

Second, he must learn to put "money" in his "bank account" and not spend every red cent that comes his way. The patient in this phase is so happy when the pall of the Exhaustion Phase is relieved that he attempts to use the false energy produced by the overstimulation of the adrenal gland by the Hypothalamic–Pituitary Axis that he rapidly uses up the little adrenal gland regeneration created by his forced rest in the Exhaustion Phase and is thus soon thrown back into this Exhaustion Phase again with little being accomplished by the small amount of adrenal gland regeneration that took place. If he is to ever master his condition, the CFS patient must learn to husband all the regenerative efforts of his adrenal gland and not to squander them on useful but destructive activities at this time in his recovery.

It was to help our patients with this phase of their cure that we instituted our live-in Sanctuary program. When patients are in our Sanctuary, we are able to reduce their need to expend energy to a minimum, and thus they are able to take advantage of this stay to build their adrenal gland bank account. We are able to monitor them daily to assure both us and them that they are not attempting to spend the energy we are building in them by our "machines" and other therapies, but are allowing it to build in their glandular bank account.

The Postural Blood Pressure test is very helpful in monitoring them during this process. As we are able to desensitize the Hypothalamic–Pituitary Axis by our treatments and remedies, we can see the blood pressure readings change from those of Hypothalamic–Pituitary Axis overstimulation (the pressures are high for the patient and rise more than 10 points upon standing) to those of adrenal gland relaxation and regeneration (the pressures are lower and there is little or no rise upon standing). If a patient allows himself to become overactive or overstimulated, we can tell it by the change in his daily blood pressure readings and are able to help him get back on the regenerative path.

There are two groups of patients that do not experience the exasperating effects of overstimulation of the adrenal gland by the Hypothalamic–Pituitary Axis. These are those patients in the first or the second Exhaustion Phases of the Selye chart. For those in the first Exhaustion Phase, the Hypothalamic–Pituitary Axis has not yet been stimulated to a state of oversensitiveness, while in the second Exhaustion Phase the adrenal gland has become so weak and exhausted that it cannot respond to even the most aggressive stimulation by the Hypothalamic–Pituitary Axis. We often have patients who come to us in a very exhausted state who assure us that they are better than they were because they used to have both exhaustion and anxiety, but now the anxiety is gone and they only have the exhaustion. Of course, they are not better, but have actually advanced into the second Exhaustion Phase where the adrenal gland is so weak that it can no longer respond to the Hypothalamic–Pituitary Axis stimulus.

Lastly, we have a group of patients who almost never seem to come out of the overstimulation by the Hypothalamic–Pituitary Axis. These individuals are anxious almost all the time. Their life is a constant torture without any of the respite of the usual anxiety-exhaustion alternation. In these patients the Hypothalamic–Pituitary Axis seems almost to have a life all its own. A phosphorylated mixture of L-Serine and Ethanolamine is the remedy for most, although occasionally we have a patient of this type that even this agent does not seem to calm down, and we must use all our tricks to help.

Summary

Long experience has taught us that a working knowledge of the interplay between the adrenal gland and the Hypothalamic–Pituitary Axis is absolutely essential for the management of the average CFS patient. Without this understanding, the symptoms of the average CFS patient seem enigmatic and illogical. I wish I had a dollar for every time a patient told me that his previous physician said that he could not possibly have the symptoms he described to me. I am able to understand the physician's disbelief, because there is to my knowledge no other condition in the medical books that displays the unique combination of exhaustion and anxiety that CFS does.

In one corner we have a valiant little adrenal gland (it weighs in about the same as a nickel) and in the other the powerful effects of the master gland (pituitary) and the brain stem (hypothalamus). While in normal body functioning these three work synergistically, in the CFS patient some very strange things begin to happen. As the actor Paul Neuman said in the movie, *Cool Hand Luke*, "What we have here is a failure to communicate."

The vast majority of true CFS symptoms can be attributed to the interplay of these two mechanisms. If the adrenal gland is weak but the Hypothalamic–Pituitary Axis is not over-stimulating it, the patient will feel exhausted. If, in the later phases of CFS, the Hypothalamic–Pituitary Axis is overactive, but the adrenal gland is too weakened to respond, we find the same nearly constant state of exhaustion in the patient.

If we have a weak adrenal gland but an overstimulation of the adrenal by the Hypothalamic–Pituitary Axis in an effort to squeeze more life out of it, we have the scenario that produces the boom-and-bust symptomatology of the common CFS patient. The Hypothalamic–Pituitary Axis cares little if the adrenal gland is exhausted or not; its job is to stimulate this gland if the hormone levels are low, and it is determined to do its duty come hell or high water. If the adrenal gland becomes too exhausted, it cannot respond to the Hypothalamic–Pituitary Axis stimulation and the patient will have a period of exhaustion; but as soon as the adrenal gland gains a little strength from the forced rest of the patient, it is again overstimulated by the Hypothalamic–Pituitary Axis. In the life of the average CFS patient in the Countershock or Resistance Phases of this condition this alternation of exhaustion and anxiety are well-known dreaded symptoms.

In some patients in the Countershock or Resistance Phases the exhaustion and anxiety do not alternate but are coincidental—a most distressing state found in no other medical condition known to me. In fact, before the ASI test became common, we often used the presence of this combination in a patient as a definitive diagnostic factor for CFS.

In a small number of CFS patients, the overstimulation of the Hypothalamic–Pituitary Axis is the predominant symptom. Most of these will respond to phosphorylated serine and ethanolamine therapy, but a few will require even more specialized therapy.

In treating the effects of the interplay of a weakened adrenal gland and an overstimulated Hypothalamic–Pituitary Axis, the patient and doctor must work very closely together. This is not a phase of CFS that is amenable to self-treatment or even to treatment by those with little experience with CFS. These patients can be helped, but the road to health is very rocky and full of pitfalls; to reach the final goal patients need the careful close monitoring of "one who knows the way."

Chapter Seven

Treatment of Chronic Fatigue Syndrome

URING our early years of treating of Chronic Fatigue Syndrome (CFS), our first efforts were to assure the patient that he had a specific condition, that its cause was known and that its correction was readily available to those who were willing to work with the doctor. This was a daunting task, and we often found the process of treating these patients much easier than convincing them that they could be treated successfully.

In the ensuing years much has changed. Today it is not as necessary to convince patients that they have a real disease, since there has been a radical change in medical thought on this subject from the time we first began to treat it. CFS is now well-known and accepted by many, if still not a majority, of family physicians. No longer are patients with this symptom pattern automatically considered neurotic or malingering. Unfortunately, the CFS patient is still as frustrated as he was before, but he has a different form of frustration. Where previously he was told, "You do not have a disease, you are only neurotic or lazy," he is now told, "You do have a disease, you have CFS, but we do not have a treatment, so you just have to learn to live with it."

In keeping with this new paradigm, we find that our main essential with our patients is no longer assuring them that they have a real physical condition, but convincing them that it can be treated successfully. After all, the old wise heads in the

119

medical hierarchy have assured them that there is no success-ful treatment. Why should they believe us to the contrary?

Fortunately, the type of person who is susceptible to CFS is almost always an intelligent, motivated individual. Once he is exposed to the logic of our approach to this condition, he is quick to grasp its logic and validity. Skepticism quickly gives way to enthusiasm to cooperate in his cure and soon he is on his way to a full recovery.

The Doctor-Patient Crusade

By the time we see most CFS patients, their condition is frequently far advanced and is going to require our most comprehensive treatment. This treatment must include life-style stress-reduction procedures. In most CFS patients it was their previous life-style that precipitated their present condi-tion, and unless changes are made for the better there is little chance of a permanent cure. I usually make it a policy to be frank with these patients and let them know early what they and I must do to conquer this condition.

In CFS, as in most other diseases to which the body is subject, the patient's success in regaining health depends as much on his attitude and cooperation as on the skill and treatment of his physician. As I will point out throughout this text, however, the nature of CFS makes it difficult for many patients to cooperate with their physician. For this reason, I sometimes impose conditions for treatment. I remember one severely ill patient whom I had refused to treat unless she stayed with us for six months of therapy. Her family fussed and fumed, but finally agreed. She returned home at the end of six months an entirely new person and remains so to this day. Had I equivocated on this case and tried less extensive treatment, I would have failed, and she would have given up long before improvement ensued.

The secret of all successful CFS therapy can be illustrated by the Classic Double-Pan Scale (Figure 1) in which the total stresses of the patient are in one pan and the total treatment in the other. If the stress pan is heavier than the treatment pan, the patient will worsen. If the treatment pan is heavier, the patient will improve, and if both are equal, the patient will remain as he is, neither getting worse nor getting better.

Figure 1 below illustrates that the amount of treatment must outweigh the force of the stresses which encumber the patient if treatment is to succeed. Therefore, successful therapy can be accomplished in three ways:

- Increase therapy until it is stronger than the stresses.

- Decrease stress so that is smaller than the therapy.

- Use methods that both increase therapy and lower stress.

An understanding of this balance mechanism allows great freedom and leeway to the type of therapy that can be applied to any individual patient. For instance, the low-income patient who cannot readily afford most of the forms of clinical therapy needed to correct his CFS can still be helped by Life Mastery counseling that will reduce the various stresses under which he lives. If the patient is able to reduce his amount of stress sufficiently so that it drops below the level of even minimal therapy, he will improve.

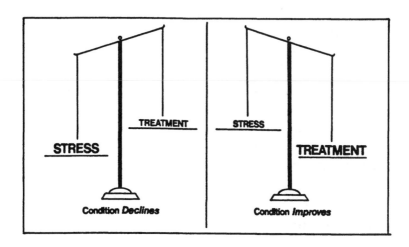

Figure 1. Classic Double-Pan Scale

At the other extreme, some patients are in such an emotional state because of their condition that it is almost impossible for them to control their external and internal stresses. These patients must come into our Clinic for complete inpatient care. Here they may receive careful personal management and an accelerated course of therapy to help support and regenerate their general adaptive mechanism. With this accelerated treatment, they will reach a point where they will be able to regain control over their internal stresses and can then return home to finish their therapy.

From the above you can see that it is entirely possible to treat two patients who are almost identical in their exposures to stress and their inherent glandular weaknesses successfully by what at first may appear to be entirely different therapy techniques. When we do this, we simply treat from opposite sides of the balance scale. In one patient, because of certain extenuating circumstances, we might concentrate on stress reduction; in another, in- or outpatient clinical treatment might be the most expeditious approach. In fact, the true skill of the physician in treating CFS is shown by knowing at all times where he needs to place the emphasis for the best healing response.

The basic mechanisms of treating CFS are simple and are fully outlined in this text. The difference between success and failure often depends on the experience and wisdom of the physician, on his knowledge of how to achieve that balance of clinical treatment and stress reduction that is best for the individual patient. Fortunately, it is not absolutely essential for most patients to have exactly the correct proportions of these two factors to improve, but the proper proportions do make for the most rapid and thorough improvement.

Specific Treatment Techniques

Specific clinical therapy can be divided into three components: internal, external, and stress counseling.

The first and foremost internal treatment is dictated by the results of the ASI test. From this test, we know the specific substances needed by the body to reestablish order and stability in the body. These remedies must be given in a certain order and in the beginning dosages that the patient can handle. Since the CFS patient has a difficult time adapting to anything new, even though it may be just what his body needs, all remedies are started in small dosages and gradually increased in dosage as the patient's ability to handle the remedy improves.

Internal treatment also includes other specific nutritional and supportive agents which are supplied to the body to aid in the regeneration of its general adaptive mechanism. It is important that the body have the substances it needs to rebuild the gland structures. If these are not available to the body, much of the other therapy is rendered ineffective.

The third component of internal therapy is diet. While there is no specific diet that is curative for CFS, a low stress-high nutrient diet is essential for a complete recovery. There are also various diets that are important in certain complications of CFS. These will be addressed later.

External methods are those treatment procedures that are utilized to regenerate the general adaptive mechanism by means that do not require any substance to enter the body. Such treatments as Magnatherm,[1] Myoflex,[2] diathermy, hydrotherapy, remedial exercises, massage, spinal corrections and tissue sludge therapy come under this classification.

The third division of clinical therapy, stress counseling, is self-explanatory. Almost all clinical therapy would be worthless if the patients were not first of all properly counseled to have an understanding and appreciation of their condition, and then trained in the methods and techniques necessary to help them to master the stresses which aggravate and prolong this problem. This is particularly important in the area of exercise and daily work effort. These two must be carefully regulated by the physician if a full recovery is to be expected.

---

[1] Manufactured by International Medical Electronics, Ltd., 2805 Main Street, Kansas City, MO 64108.

[2] Originally manufactured by M. J. Edwards, 3515 Velva St., Shreveport, LA 71109.

Internal Therapies

The Adrenal Stress Index Specifics

There are only so many things that can be shown to be needed by the ASI test to rebalance the neurohormonal system of the body. The basic ones are: Dr. Baschetti's pure licorice extract, DHEA, pregnenolone and a phosphorylated mixture of L-Serine and Ethanolamine. If the ASI reveals a depressed immune system, as it frequently does, then we must add thymic extract, EMP™ and other immune support to this list.

Dr. Baschetti's pure licorice extract, along with some of the nutritional remedies mentioned below, is given to the CFS patient whose morning cortisol levels are below normal.

DHEA is given to most men who show a need for this hormone precursor on their ASI test results, while pregnenolone is used to do the same thing in women as DHEA does in men. DHEA may be given to women, but it does tend to cause some effects of female hormone overdose such as tender breasts. Since pregnenolone seems to have the same benefits for women as DHEA does for men (minus the side effects), we prefer it for women in our Clinic rather than DHEA.

The phosphorylated mixture of L-Serine and Ethanolamine is the remedy best suited at the present time to help control the oversensitivity of the Hypothalamic–Pituitary Axis. We use a product, designed by those who discovered the effectiveness of the phosphorylated mixture of L-Serine and Ethanolamine in regulating the Hypothalamic–Pituitary Axis. From the CFS patient's ASI test, the status of this Hypothalamic–Pituitary Axis can be determined and the amount and timing of this remedy prescribed accordingly.

Perhaps the most distressing symptom of those with an overactive Hypothalamic–Pituitary Axis is various forms of insomnia. Some patients have trouble getting to sleep, some have trouble staying asleep (they wake up several times during the night from the adrenaline being dumped into the system by the overactive Hypothalamic–Pituitary Axis), and some have both symptoms. The phosphorylated mixture of L-Serine and Ethanolamine is effective in ameliorating all these symptoms.

The dosage of this mixture must be carefully managed. As with all other remedies for CFS patients, we start with a small dose and gradually build it up. In some patients the dose may need to go as high as ten to twelve capsules a day before the sleep symptoms are corrected. Even then it may take some time to relieve these symptoms if the CFS is well entrenched.

When we find the immune system depressed we add thymic extract, EMP™ or similar remedies to the patient's program. These are dedicated to supporting and normalizing the immune system. They help the body to fight off infections and inflammations until the immune system can be regenerated by the balancing of the glandular system.

Nutritional Supplements

Once the patient's specific ASI test requirements are met, we are ready to look into his general nutritional therapy. Proper supplemental therapy is probably the single most important clinical treatment component in the mild to moderate case. Without this therapy, it is rare for true and permanent improvement in the CFS patient. It alone is sufficient to make dramatic improvement in many of the milder cases. In our Centers, we usually use a supplement containing vitamin C, calcium pantothenate, vitamin B-6, citrus bioflavinoids, zinc (complexed with amino acids from rice) and raw concentrates of adrenal, spleen and thymus. This last compound, which is absolutely essential to proper adrenal regeneration, is made by desiccating bovine gland material at below body temperature so as not to destroy any of the delicate RNA and DNA factors necessary to help supply these glands with the nutrients they need for regeneration. This product was designed to our specifications and has proven its worth over two decades.

Occasionally, we use other products for patients who are sensitive to the fairly high doses of vitamin C contained in the previously mentioned product. We often need to use remedies that contain only the raw adrenal concentrate. There are several such remedies we always keep on hand to satisfy the sensitivities of our CFS patients.

In the last few years, many nutritional supplement producers have introduced compounds allegedly designed to help regenerate the neurohormonal mechanism. We feel that some of this interest is due to our pioneering work in creating an increased awareness to CFS. However, the only products for whose integrity we can personally vouch for are those used in our Centers. This is not to intimate that some of these other products may not be of help, only that I have not had sufficient experience with any them to make a recommendation. Our experience has shown that it is not sufficient to merely capsule adrenal gland substance and purport to have a product to aid in the regeneration of the CFS patient. Many vital factors in these substances are easily destroyed by improper extraction or careless manufacturing procedures. At this time we have no way of analyzing for certain whether these newer products contain the elements that will help CFS patients or not. Only through long clinical experience can this information be ascertained. Because of this fact, please do not judge the effectiveness of the treatment recommended in this text unless you are using the specific compounds that we have tested. They are the only ones we know for certain will work.

Next to the adrenal gland substance supplement, I find the elements of the vitamin B-complex family most vital. The compound that has proven the most effective for us is derived from a combination of natural sources: yeast, liver, and rice-bran concentrates. This product contains many of the coenzymes that in my experience are essential to proper adrenal regeneration and are not usually contained in purified formulations. This product also contains additional glandular extracts to help provide the multiple glandular support of the general adaptive mechanism. Thus, we are providing the plural-glandular technique so much favored by Dr. Henry Harrower in his work, *Practical Organic Therapy, The Internal Secre-*

tions in General Practice. I have not yet found an effective substitute for this agent, therefore, cannot recommend any other product as having the same beneficial effect for the CFS patient.

Where more substantial nutritional support is needed, we recommend a variety of nutritional support. While we may attempt to do so from the patient's history, we prefer that a more specific determination of the patient's needs is made.

If the CFS patient is able to afford an in-depth analysis of his specific supplemental needs without creating a burdensome financial stress, we recommend a group of screening tests that we developed many years ago when I was Director of the Clymer Health Clinic. We term these tests Specific Nutritional Profile. In this procedure, special examinations of the blood, urine, hair and diet are made, which provide us with a detailed report of the patient's individual body's deficiencies and imbalances. Following the completion of this testing procedure, it is a simple matter to suggest the specific diet and/ or nutritional substances needed to aid in rebalancing the body's chemistries. In moderate to severe CFS cases such procedures are absolutely essential.

To understand the need for such balancing of the body, we must once again return to the analogy shown in Figure 1. Any reduction in his stress helps the CFS patient recover more rapidly. By analyzing his body's chemistry and creating optimal nutritional balance within his system, one very important form of stress is reduced—this can be essential with certain patients and useful with all.

Adrenal Cortical Extract[3]

In previous editions of this book we wrote a great deal about adrenal cortical extract. It was one of the mainstays of

---

[3] Adrenal cortical extract differs from the raw adrenal concentrates in that, unlike them, it contains the various normal hormones present in the cortex of the adrenal gland. It is not used to supply nutrients to the cells of the adrenal gland, as do the raw adrenal concentrates, but to actually supply adrenal cortical hormones to the bloodstream.

our treatment of the CFS patient. Unfortunately, the availability of this substance engendered the ire of some of the large drug companies who produced synthetic steroid products. While adrenal cortical extract (ACE) took very few profits away from these large companies, it was apparently enough to have them entreat the Food and Drug Administration (FDA) to remove this product from the market.

The FDA soon discovered that this request was not as easily carried out as it seemed at first. ACE had been on the market for many years and there were no incidences of adverse effects or dangers to the public. It was far safer than aspirin and had been on the market almost as long as this drug. Finally, some smart minion of the FDA got the bright idea to call it an "obsolete drug." Since no one was quite certain what this Gilbert-and-Sullivan-style term meant for sure, the FDA officials were able to establish their own definition and consequences. These protectors of our safety determined that the synthetic products of the big drug companies had made the use of ACE "obsolete" and therefore it would not be allowed on the market any longer, thus, forcing every doctor to use the synthetic products of their good friends (and often, future employers) the large entrenched international drug cartel.

The only way that ACE could legitimately be marketed in the future would be if some manufacturer would apply to the FDA for a "New Drug" application for this substance. This process costs many millions of dollars and is only practical if the product, once approved, can be patented so that the company can recoup its research and development cost and make a little (or a lot of) profit. This patent process was not possible with ACE, since it was not in actuality a "New Drug," but a very well-known and long-trusted part of medicine. For this reason no manufacturer has attempted, or will attempt, to apply for a "New Drug" application for ACE. Thus we see how, by a cute semantic subterfuge, the FDA was able to stay on the good side of the drug cartel and deprive all CFS patients of an important remedy for their regeneration and cure.

For a time after the FDA debacle we were able to get some

good dependable ACE from other countries, particularly from Germany and Italy. But soon the long tentacles of the international drug cartel squeezed these sources dry as well.

Our last source of injectable ACE was from small "underground" companies who were making it illegally in the USA. While some of this supply was good, some was contaminated and could cause serious injury to several patients. Since we do not know of any ACE injectable product at this time that is guaranteed to be safe, we no longer use this product in our treatment of CFS.

Despite all the above, we still believe that there is an important place for ACE in the treatment of CFS. At the present time we are using a sublingual (under-the-tongue) ACE with good effect. Since it is not injected this product may be sold as a nutritional supplement. We have had no problems with this form of administration and its effectiveness approaches that of the injectable substance. The sublingual ACE is used similarly to the injectable form in that it is used by us to rest the adrenal gland, thereby encouraging its regeneration rather than attempting to supplant the hormones of the body's own glandular system.

The following indented paragraphs on ACE were found in my original text, *Adrenal Syndrome*. They are retained here because they still are pertinent to the treatment of CFS with the sublingual ACE and with other methods designed to "shut off" the adrenal glands so that they are able to regenerate. Also there is always the hope that some day the iron grip of the international drug cartel on the American public will be relaxed and we may again be able to obtain a safe and effective injectable ACE at a moderate cost.

> Once the dietary and supplemental requirements of the patient are met, one rather controversial form of internal therapy remains. That is, the use of adrenal cortical extract (ACE) injections. Other injectable agents have proven useful in the treatment of CFS, and they will be discussed here also. To understand

the value as well as the possible misuse of adrenal cortical extract, we must review the functioning of the adrenal glands in these patients.

In normal functioning, the adrenal glands work similarly to that of a thermostatically controlled furnace. When the heat in the home drops below a certain level, the furnace starts and continues until the temperature rises to a certain predetermined level, at which point the furnace shuts itself off and remains off until the temperature again reaches the thermostatically controlled lower-level setting at which the furnace again turns on. In the properly functioning furnace, this procedure is carried on ad infinitum as weather and outside temperature require. The adrenal glands, as well as most other endocrine glands of the body, are controlled by a similar mechanism. The body requires for its general functioning a certain level of cortical hormones. Normal adrenal glands release these hormonal substances into the bloodstream when the level in the blood reaches a point below which the body can function optimally. The adrenal glands continue to secrete these substances until a certain preset level is reached, at which point, like the furnace, they shut off, not to resume secretion until the hormones in the bloodstream reach the previously mentioned low point again. Then, as the furnace, they begin to secrete anew and continue to repeat this process as need arises.

We now know that there is another functioning mechanism involved that has to be considered in this matter and that is the Hypothalamic–Pituitary Axis mentioned in the previous chapter. While the mechanism described above functions on a constant basis, there is also an emergency override in place in the body. This is the Hypothalamic–Pituitary Axis. This axis comes into action if there is need for an extra supply of adrenal hormones to meet emergencies. When this axis is stimulated by the needs of the body (fear, fright, danger, etc.), it will stimulate the adrenal gland to pour out an extra dose of hormones into the blood.

For those CFS patients in the Countershock or Resistance Phases of CFS the Hypothalamic–Pituitary Axis becomes oversensitive, and every little incident can induce the weakened adrenal to pour out what little hormones it contains. While in our experience the ACE does have some effect on controlling the Hypothalamic–Pituitary Axis (as do the passive office treatments we give at our Center), the phosphorylated mixture of L-Serine and Ethanolamine is the main agent we now use to control the oversensitivity of this mechanism.

There are two basic ways in which ACE may be used to help the CFS patient. The first is as a massive replacement therapy to augment regular adrenal functioning. The second technique is to use it to allow rest periods for the adrenal glands so that they may regenerate. In the first instance, large amounts of ACE—from 10cc to 20cc—are injected into the venous system once or twice a week. Many doctors have in the past used this procedure with some success for treating hypoglycemia. (My own feeling is that they were actually treating the low adrenal functioning which many feel is one of the main causes of hypoglycemia.)

Large Dosages of ACE

The injection of large amounts of adrenal cortical extract into the venous system can be therapeutically dramatic and may be essential in certain severe, acute states of CFS. But for the average chronic patient under long-term care it has certain drawbacks, which I feel negate its usefulness. I do not feel that it is physiologically sound therapy for chronic cases. As mentioned earlier, all endocrine glands are stimulated by a demand mechanism. That is, they are stimulated to secrete when the blood levels of their hormones reach a certain low point and to shut off when these levels reach another somewhat higher point. If massive amounts of a gland's secretions are given to the body on a regular basis, the gland will be inhibited to such an extent that it will stop producing adequate amounts of its own secretions. This is basic human physiology. If large amounts of ACE are continually pumped into a patient's bloodstream, he will feel better, it is true, and the adrenal glands will be shut off and allowed to rest. This in itself is beneficial, but if injection of these amounts is continued, the gland no longer has a need to produce its own secretions. The demand mechanism will not trigger because of the high levels of ACE in the bloodstream. If this high dosage of ACE is continued for an extended period of time, the adrenal gland possibly could reach a state in which it can no longer regenerate.[4] While this

---

[4] Nowadays there is very little chance of ACE being used in this manner since it is almost unobtainable (and that which is obtainable is not recommended), but in its place doctors are using the synthetic pharmaceuticals such as Cortef® and Florinef®. These not only will depress the natural adrenal hormones, as do large doses of ACE, but add to this adverse effect the many serious side effects of cortisone on the body. In our own practice we put patients on the synthetic steroids only during obvious emergencies. However, we spend a great deal of time and effort getting patients off steroids that have been prescribed by previous physicians.

may not occur in every case, and may not occur as often as we fear, we are meddling with a delicate balance when we use ACE in this manner.

Another problem with the intravenous injection of ACE is that it makes the patient too dependent on the doctor. In our work, we attempt to make our patients as independent as possible. Only by building up their confidence in themselves and their own abilities as individuals can we truly reduce and keep minimal the various stresses they must confront as functioning human beings. The more they depend on other individuals, even their doctor, the more difficult it is to reach this state.

Another not-to-be forgotten factor is the high cost of adrenal cortical extract; it is not an inexpensive remedy, and used in such large amounts can be an inordinate financial drain on the CFS patient. I personally recommend this procedure only for a patient who is overwhelmed by unremitting stress from which he cannot extricate himself due to factors not under his own personal control and for whom all other methods of therapy have not been adequate to tip the scales in his favor. In twenty-five years [now forty-one] of treating this condition, I fortunately have found few patients who fell into this extreme category. Even in these few severe instances, the patients were kept on the massive dosage for only a short time. As soon as possible the patient was placed on the lower dosage ACE and/or oral therapy. Patients with such severe symptoms might well be treated with a cortisone preparation by an orthodox practitioner; while I am not enamored with the use of large dosages of ACE, it is far less toxic than the cortisone compounds.

There is one other time at which large doses of ACE have been found helpful—in the differential diagnosis of CFS from those conditions which may mimic it. If the true CFS patient is given an injection of 10cc to 20cc of 2-x ACE, he should notice considerable improvement in his entire being within a few minutes to hours. This improvement should last a day or two at least, and then gradually subside. Should the patient notice no improvement from this amount of ACE, the adrenal component of his problem is probably not the major cause of his symptoms and the health professional should look to food allergies, defects in brain nutrition, hypoglycemia, hypothyroidism or some other related difficulty for his main problem.[5]

Low Dose Usage of ACE

In our Clinic, we have perfected a low-dosage use of adrenal cortical extract (ACE) that seems to overcome the difficulties encountered with the large-dosage intravenous method and is capable of providing practically all of the therapeutic value of the large dose. This is especially true for the chronic case. As used in our Clinic, the purpose of the adrenal cortical extract is not to supplant the secretions of the person's own glands, but as a method of permitting the

---

[5] At this time therapeutic tests may be run with hydrocortisone (Cortef® or Florinef®). Since the drug is only used for a few days at most, there is no time for the adverse side effects or adrenal inhibition to endanger the patient. The patient must be informed, of course, that this use of the synthetic steroid is only for diagnostic purposes and will not be used for treatment.

adrenal glands to rest and regenerate. I stress this point because many patients expect to feel better as soon as they start to receive the injections, only to discover that they are sometimes more exhausted and less capable of pushing themselves than they were before this treatment started. This is the desired result and is easily explained if we examine the physiology of the patient. With these injections, we attempt to raise the level of the adrenal cortical hormones in the blood to the point at which the adrenal glands shut off for a period of rest. This is essential for adrenal recovery, because only during periods when the adrenal glands are at rest are they capable of regeneration. There is no chance of improvement for the CFS patient who does not obtain these important periods of adrenal rest. At times, the exhaustion following the first ACE shots persists which is explainable by the fact that once a gland that has been running a long time without rest shuts off, it is often difficult for it to start up again. It is like an individual who has gone several days without sleep; once he goes to sleep, he may sleep for an inordinately long time and be difficult to arouse.

The adrenal glands so need this rest that often the levels of the hormone in the blood drop below the normal turn-on point before this resting gland reactivates itself. During this period in which the blood levels of the cortical hormones are low, the patient feels much more tired and exhausted than usual. It can be a good exhaustion, however. By that I mean an exhaustion without the anxiety which is produced by the constantly running weakened adrenal glands and the elevated levels of cortisol and adrenaline.[6] Unfortunately, all too many Chronic Fatigue Syndrome patients expect a rapid and uneventful recovery and consider a treatment good only if it produces in them what they call a normal feeling, that is, the feeling that is present with fully functioning adrenal hormones in the blood. This feeling can and will come to every adrenal patient who is treated properly, but it does not usually come by proper therapeutic use of adrenal cortical extract alone.

Not all patients respond to ACE with this state of increased exhaustion. In fact, the degree of depth of CFS is often indicated by the patient's reaction to small amounts of ACE. If the patient feels a lift from an injection, I consider the case mild and easy to cure because the level of hormone is near normal and the addition of a small amount of ACE raised his hormonal level to a degree sufficient to create a symptomatic improvement.

Patients who notice no real effect from ACE injections—and these are the great majority— are considered to be moderately severe. In these patients, the adrenal hormone is low enough so that the addition of a small amount of ACE in the body does not make sufficient change to produce an immediate alleviation of the symptoms. On the other hand, the adrenal gland is not so weakened that it cannot respond by "coming on line" once the level of body hormones drops to the turn-on point.

---

[6] While the action of the Hypothalamic–Pituitary Axis is to stimulate the adrenal gland to produce cortisol and not the medullary hormone adrenaline, there is usually some spillover stimulation of this medullary hormone with the symptoms so typical of an adrenaline rush.

When a patient experiences increased exhaustion after receiving ACE, we consider his case to be more serious because his adrenals are not capable of readily resuming activity when the hormone levels are below this turn-on point.

ACE is most often given in dosages ranging from 1cc to 4cc, using the 2-x variety. Injections are given daily in serious cases to as infrequently as once a month in those patients who are well on the road to recovery.[7]

Not all CFS patients require ACE, and our general clinical policy is to treat the patient by the most natural, least harmful and most inexpensive approach possible. Over the years, as we have become known for our treatment of this condition, we attract more of the serious, chronic-type patients, and in these instances ACE is frequently a vital factor in their recovery.

Certain other injectable substances have been found to be beneficial when given in conjunction with ACE. These include such nutritional compounds as a calcium-phosphorus compound, vitamin B-12, vitamin B-6, vitamin B-1 and raw crude liver.[8]

---

[7] When we use the sublingual ACE, it too is given daily in doses that fit the needs of the patient. We usually begin with a few drops and build up the dosage to the patient's optimum as determined by his response. While it is often possible to obtain oral ACE from health food stores, it is not recommended that an individual attempt to use this substance unless he is being monitored by a physician who knows how to manage a patient on ACE. ACE in not something you take as a general supplement. It has a very special use at a certain time in the care of some CFS patients. It should never be used unless it is advised by a physician after he has made an ASI test.

[8] Today these are often given at our Woodlands Healing Research Center in the form of an intravenous drip. This is used on those patients who do not readily respond to our usual oral medication.

Diet

Every CFS patient wants us to give him a diet that will cure his condition. There is no such thing, and I can assure him of this from long experience with this condition. On the other hand a poor diet can do much to keep a patient from getting better. Therefore, diet of the CFS patient is important; it's just that it is not curative by itself.

We generally recommend a low-stress diet which provides, in as readily assimilable form as possible, all of the nutrient elements needed for satisfactory bodily function with special emphasis on those compounds that help to regenerate the general adaptive mechanism. The diet should be arranged to include only the foods that are most easily digested, absorbed and metabolized. It should exclude all foods that contain toxic substances that place added stress on the system and foods that require more energy to digest and assimilate than they return to the body in nutritive value. For the patient who does not have frank hypoglycemia, I usually use a combination of our Clinic's Basic Health Maintenance Diet and the Hypoglycemic Diet. (See Appendix I for diets.) The frequent meals, moderate protein and increased intake of fruits and vegetables of the Hypoglycemic Diet seem to fit the needs of most CFS patients. In general, we allow most of our CFS patients to have reasonable amounts of honey, dried fruits, rice, bananas, potatoes, and other starchy foods that are usually excluded from the diet of true hypoglycemic patients.

The foods chosen should be as free of pesticides and additives as possible. Although organically grown foods are not an absolute prerequisite, we find that patients who are able to obtain and use organically grown foods or their homegrown counterparts recover more rapidly. Attempts should also be made to obtain chicken, fish, lean meat and other proteins from as reliable a source as possible. Try to get them as fresh and free from chemical additives as possible, since such chemicals are still being used in many of these products.

When the general adaptive mechanism begins to fail, one of the first body functions to be impeded is the digestive system. Therefore, most of these patients have digestive problems to a lesser or greater degree, and it is all the more important that every mouthful of food these patients take be as nutritious and non-stress-producing as possible.

While the digestive mechanism is usually affected in most CFS patients, it may be affected in different and sometimes diametrically opposite ways in individual patients. In some, the condition called anorexia, or poor appetite, is present. These patients must be supplied with small but frequent amounts of highly nutritious foods. In others, the appetite becomes voracious, as if the body were attempting to make up in quantity what it lacks in quality. The new gastric analysis instrument, known as the Heidelberg pH monitoring instrument,[9] can be of great help in determining imbalances present in the individual patient's digestive system and in providing specific information as to what form of supplementation is needed to overcome his digestive dysfunctioning. Having this information is important, because in the healthy individual there is a balance of hydrochloric acid and the acidic-working enzymes of the stomach, the alkaline-working enzymes of the duodenum and small intestine, the fat-emulsifying elements from the gall bladder and the bacterial breakdown of foods in the large intestine.

Normal digestion requires a proper synchronization of all of these factors. With the failure of the general adaptive mechanism, this synchronization frequently becomes disturbed. These patients are best helped by a rebalancing of this synchronization so that foods and supplements may be utilized to their best advantage. Many CFS patients have great difficulty digesting and absorbing the specific supplements that are essential to improvement of their condition. For these patients, it is necessary to work on the digestive system before the internal portion of the clinical treatment can be instituted in a proper manner.

---

[9] Manufactured by AEG-Telefunken, West Germany. Distributed by ElectroMedical Devices, Inc., Scientific Instruments Division, 6669 Peachtree Industrial Boulevard, Atlanta, GA 30092.

The Heidelberg pH monitoring instrument mentioned before is extremely helpful in determining digestive system synchronization. With this diagnostic instrument, a special miniaturized radio transmitter and pH meter, no larger than a vitamin pill, is ingested and monitored by a special receiver-recorder as it passes through the digestive system. This little capsule sends out harmless radio signals to an instrument which graphs the changes in pH as it passes through the stages of digestion. The synchronous nature of the digestive system can be evaluated quite accurately by knowing the time intervals and the pH, that is, the degree of acid or alkaline, at any specific time as the transmitter traverses the digestive tract. From this knowledge, the degree and nature of the digestive imbalance can be calculated and necessary measures taken to correct it. This correction is accomplished by the use of various digestants, special food combinations, and therapy directed to the nerve centers in control of digestion.

Many patients with Chronic Fatigue Syndrome also have various food sensitivities. In these patients, even the best of regular diets can be injurious. Special testing must be done to ascertain the patient's needs. These procedures are described in a later chapter.

External Clinical Treatment

The most misunderstood and unappreciated part of the treatment of CFS is the external clinical treatment. It is not difficult to explain to a patient suffering from this complaint how various stress-reducing procedures are going to help him. Most of us are accustomed to taking pills and injections, and we have little difficulty in understanding how this type of therapy is going to help. But many find it difficult to understand how a machine can help regenerate their adrenal glands. Nevertheless, the external treatment is usually a must for speedy recovery, and as the years go by we find that it is most often the main treatment we have that helps us to regenerate patients after all other help has failed.

"The Machines"

The two most useful machines (I like to call them "regenerative therapy instruments," but my patients insist on calling them "the machines") we use are the Magnatherm and the Myoflex (see footnotes on page 123). They have a similar purpose, although they work on entirely different principles. The Magnatherm produces a pulsating electromagnetic energy, while the Myoflex effects a complex multiple sine-wave current which is designed to mimic the electrical impulse energy produced by the human nerve cell.

Before I go into detail about these two instruments, I wish to mention other methods of external treatment. If muscle tension and spasm have been produced from long-encountered bodily stress, the standard diathermy and/or sine-wave machines are often helpful in reducing this problem. When muscle tension is accompanied by nervous irritation, such external therapies as the whirlpool bath, sauna, wet-sheet pack and various forms of massage are extremely helpful. All these are effective, predicated on an understanding of the basic premise stated at the beginning of this chapter, *i.e.*, any form of treatment that produces a reduction of stress in the body, mind or soul relieves the general adaptive system, and, therefore, helps the CFS patient to improve.

In the last few years we have added a new therapy to those mentioned above—the Microlight 830 low light laser. It is useful in mitigating the aches and pains (called fibromyalgia by most physicians) that often complicate CFS. It is amazing how many times the Microlight 830 will take away such a troublesome pain almost instantly.

We are also using the Microlight 830 on the nerve roots that feed the adrenal gland to see if this will help seed the regeneration of this gland and our early results are most encouraging.

While the Magnatherm and the Myoflex may seem at first to be similar to the other therapies I have just discussed, the basic mechanism of their functioning is different. The purpose of the Magnatherm and Myoflex treatments is not to reduce stress on the body; it is actually to encourage the regeneration of the bodily organs. These instruments, in my experience, have the capability of helping to regenerate organs and tissues that are not, under the present state of the CFS patient's body, able to regenerate themselves. In our Clinic, we treat the liver, spleen, adrenals, kidneys and the abdominal digestive system. This method encompasses a great deal of the reticuloendothelial system and helps to mobilize the general adaptive system. Can I prove that they work? I only know that for the past forty-one years I have been constantly refining the treatment of this condition. Many therapies have been tried; many therapies have been discarded. The ones I use now have stood the test of time. We have tried our therapy with and without the "machines," and that with the machines wins hands down every time; no contest.

Some Chronic Fatigue Sydrome patients with severe allergic sensitivities are not able to take our usual internal medication without severe reactions. The only clinical therapy possible for these allergic patients is "the machines." These trustworthy servants have never yet let me down. Usually after a short time on the machines the patient improves sufficiently to be able to begin internal treatment and go on to ultimate recovery.

From time to time a patient does not make the progress we expect, and I am concerned, because with the therapy and counseling he receives, he should be better. Almost invariably, upon querying him about the machine treatment, I have found that due to lack of time on his part, or more generally due to a misunderstanding of the value of these treatments, he has not been taking the recommended Myoflex and Magnatherm treatments. Once these treatments again become a regular part of his therapy, his progress returns to a normal rate. We feel the Magnatherm and Myoflex both work by directing the healing forces of the body to specific areas of need. They also have an effect on the electronic nature of the cell, and through this influence stimulate cellular regeneration. Such cell-level regeneration is difficult to prove, however, so we let the results speak for themselves.[10]

Manual Therapies

It's been my observation that most hypoadrenal cases also have nerve-muscle-bone displacements and tensions in the area of the shoulder blade and along the upper thoracic and lower neck areas.

These we treat with mild ultrasound therapy and with finger pressure, working the sensitive areas to gradually eliminate the nerve-muscle spasms and in turn any bony displacements. In some of the more sensitive patients, this work must be handled with great delicacy; but as improvement occurs the pressure may be increased. In fact, we find that as the adrenal condition of our patient improves, he becomes less and less sensitive to this treatment and he finds it increasingly more pleasant. Now that the Microlight 830 low light laser is available, we use this delectable new therapy on these spots as well.

The explanation for the relief from soreness in the upper back and neck that patients receive from this simple maneuver is simple. When the glandular system is low, lactic acid and other acid metabolites tend to accumulate in the muscle areas of the shoulder and upper back. The ultrasound, low light laser therapy and finger pressure break up these acid deposits so they are free to return to the circulating blood to be eliminated from the body by the usual routes of elimination. While this is an apparently simple component of our therapy, many patients find it a very important one. I particularly recall two patients, a mother and her daughter, whom I had been treating for some time without the success we desired. The treatment had been long, but results slow due to a constant, unremitting stress factor at home that could simply not be

---

[10] In this edition of *Chronic Fatigue Unmasked 2000*, we are including, in Appendix IV, the chapter on the Magnatherm and related instruments from our book, *It's Only Natural* . That chapter will give all CFS patients the background on this subject that they may desire.

changed or improved. At one time in their treatment, however, I noticed—by the look in their eyes—that they both seemed to be going downhill. At that time, I sat down with them and went over every component of their treatment. They were taking all of the forms of internal therapies; they were taking the machine therapies regularly; and they were coming to the clinic twice a week, that was even more than I had asked. The only thing that they were not doing was getting the tissue sludge massage therapy, because they thought it would prolong their visits. I persuaded them to start this part of the therapy once again to see if it would help with their improvement. With the first treatment they felt better. By the end of two weeks, they were nearly back to their old selves. Since the stress at home had not changed, I continued to see them as patients. But they remained in a much improved condition, and were thereafter certain to get their full manipulative and massage therapies each visit.

Spinal manipulation, while different from the tissue sludge technique described above, has always proven to be a useful and important part of our clinical treatment of this syndrome. It has several factors going for it. It can be a great reducer of both physical and emotional stress. Both emotional and mental stress produce tension in the body's physical structures. This tension manifests itself most commonly around the neck, shoulders and back areas. All of these areas are intimately associated with the spine and its adjacent structures. By freeing this physical manifestation of the patient's tension, there is a reduction in the tendency for his nervous stress to continuously reproduce itself by the following mechanism. If we become upset or tense through some nervous stress or tension, our physical structure may go into spasm, which produces tension on the nerves and other allied soft tissues. Such physical tension can reduce a patient's basic feeling of well-being. This makes him more susceptible to nervous and emotional stress, which, in turn, produces more physical stress, which, in turn, further reduces his well-being, producing a vicious circle which must be broken somewhere along its course to enable him to feel well again.

One of the simplest and most productive methods of restoring the patient's feeling of well-being is to break up the physical tensions that occur in the body. This is one of the most important results from all forms of manipulative therapies—tissue sludge massage, deep-muscle treatments, chiropractic therapies and even various exercise programs. The now-popular jogging and running procedures also have a somewhat similar effect, although they are not as specific as the use of spinal manipulation and deep massage and are not usually recommended for CFS patients, since they would be an overstress for most of them.

Medical opinion to the contrary, there are such things as vertebral subluxations, that is, spinal segments out of alignment. This misalignment can be a primary cause of physical stresses, and the only way that these can be reduced is by spinal manipulation. Many patients with CFS cannot obtain full recovery until certain spinal misalignments are corrected by a series of spinal manipulations.

Various forms of massage, hydrotherapy and other therapies in use at our Centers fall into the category of stress-reducing external techniques. They all have their place. Their effectiveness in each case varies with the nature of the individual. Sometimes half an hour with our massage therapist helps some patients to relax when nothing else seems to do so. Other CFS patients do not want to be touched by anyone, and the same massage therapy which was so efficacious for one patient will create severe tension in another. There is no specific detailed therapeutic protocol that fits every CFS patient. There are basic guidelines, however, which must be followed: Reduce all forms of stress as much as possible and then support and regenerate the general adaptive mechanism. The methods by which these two goals are accomplished in any individual case must always be left to the discernment and discrimination of the doctor handling that patient. To paraphrase an old proverb: "One patient's relaxation is another patient's stress."

Perhaps it is this very inability to prescribe a specific useful treatment for each patient with this condition that has made the disease so difficult to recognize and accept by most practitioners. It may be why they prefer not to accept such cases. As we mentioned previously, a patient from Pittsburgh, Pennsylvania, who had a severe case of adrenal exhaustion, asked me to find a doctor nearer his home. I gave him names of several doctors who I knew had the ability to treat his disease, but in each instance, as soon as the physician discovered the patient had CFS, he refused to accept him as a patient.

Summary

The first step in the clinical treatment of CFS is to assure the patient that he has a specific condition which can be treated. In dealing with CFS, another important factor is to reduce stress—emotional, mental and physical—through integrated use of internal and external therapies and therapeutic counseling. In internal treatment, attention is given to diet and to nutritional supplements, both devised specifically for each individual patient. Special attention is given to those remedies that are dictated from the results of the ASI test. External treatment includes manual therapy and use of instruments. Therapeutic counseling, described in the next chapter, like the other treatment techniques, is individually oriented and is one of the most important aspects of the treatment regime. Throughout the patient's entire program of regaining health and stability he must be accepting of his condition and make an effort to progress one step at a time.

Chapter Eight

Life-Style Counseling for CFS

"He that won't be counseled, can't be helped."
—Benjamin Franklin.

NE of the most vital treatments for the Chronic Fatigue Syndrome (CFS) patient is life-style counseling. Before we can fully appreciate the importance and value of counseling for CFS patients, we need to visualize what has usually happened to these patients before they come under our therapy. Strange and enigmatic symptoms began to develop and then gradually intensified in these individuals. They sought help from this doctor and that doctor, from this psychologist and that psychologist, trying to find an answer to problems. Usually, each professional gave them a different answer. In each instance a different therapy was tried, with little or no improvement. Many sufferers were assured during these periods that they had a mental difficulty. Most have tried so many different therapies without real success that by the time they come to us they are ready to accept a diagnosis of mental illness and are afraid to expect improvement for fear of once again having their hopes dashed. Their friends and relatives are eager to give them advice, none of which seems to help—in fact, all of which seems to depress them further. They are in truth the emotional dregs of society. Their self-confidence and emotional stability, on a scale of one to ten, usually are at a minus six. If ever patients are in need of counseling and

some kind words, CFS patients are the ones.[1]

Once our diagnosis is finalized, life-style counseling should begin. Several specific objectives are to be achieved through counseling, the first and foremost of which is to explain his condition to the patient. Before he can be helped, the patient must accept the diagnosis and understand the character of CFS. It is imperative that he realize that it is a physical condition which, even though it may have been with him for many years, is treatable and correctable. Strange to say, as good as this news is, it is difficult for most people to accept. They usually are locked into one of two diametrically opposite patterns of thought. In one group are persons who are unwilling to accept that they have a type of condition that requires a lengthy and complicated treatment. They vainly hope that it is merely a vitamin or mineral deficiency which, once detected and corrected, will let them become their old selves once again in a few days. At the other end of the spectrum are those who are positive that the condition is really a mental disease or of such a nature that it is untreatable, so there is no real hope for them. The truth, of course, lies somewhere in between. It is the obligation and duty of the doctor who really wants to cure CFS to constantly reiterate this fact until the patient truly understands and accepts the nature of the condition and the treatment needed for recovery.

In the first instance, the patients constantly say to themselves, "There's nothing really that much wrong with me. I've just got some little problem that is making me tired. If I just get enough rest, I'll be all right again; if I can just find that right

---

[1] This was written fifteen years ago, long before the diagnosis of CFS had been coined, much less accepted. While the orthodox view of these patients today is quite different from what it was fifteen years ago, the emotional outlook for them has improved little. Now instead of saying you're crazy, the doctors say "You've got CFS, but there is no treatment or cure." In some ways it was easier for the CFS patient to accept the "crazy" diagnosis, because at least there are some cures for this diagnosis. So we see the more things change with the orthodox view of CFS, the more they stay the same. Now more than ever these patients need dedicated life-style counseling to get better.

vitamin or that missing mineral, or if some doctor would give me the right adjustment, then I'll be better." They expect a cure without any real effort on their part. Patients of this first group are not willing to accept the condition mainly because such acceptance requires them to acknowledge a degree of problem they wish to deny. Such acceptance requires a change in their life habits and a certain amount of dedication to overcome the difficulty. It is hard for many to accept that they have certain hereditary weaknesses of their glandular systems, but until they do, there can be no real help for them—in our Clinic or elsewhere. Many times patients whom I diagnosed as having CFS left unconvinced, to seek other opinions, only to return months or years later in far worse condition. They were at last willing to accept my diagnosis, having failed to find help elsewhere. Unfortunately, they then were much more difficult to help because the condition had considerably progressed.

Patients in the second category usually readily accept the fact that they have the condition. But their attitude often is, "Oh, I probably have it all right, but I know I'll never get over it." The situation is right back where it started, because the whole purpose of getting patient acceptance is to obtain patient cooperation for treatment, and these patients have given up before they started. Without patient cooperation, any treatment is long and protracted, because for adequate response the patient must realize what he has, accept what he has, acknowledge that the treatment can overcome the condition and work with the doctor toward this end. It is the counselor's job to convince these patients that they can be helped.

Once patient acceptance has been achieved, special counseling is begun to reduce emotional and psychological stresses that are present in the patient. This procedure can be one of the most time-consuming, grueling and yet rewarding procedures involved in the treatment of CFS.

Types of Stress

There are three basic types of stress which the patient can manifest. The first is physical stress; the second, mental stress;

and the third, emotional stress. The least damaging is physical stress; next comes mental stress, and the most harmful and far reaching is emotional stress. In our counseling sessions we deal mainly with mental and emotional stress.

Many patients ask how to differentiate between mental stress and emotional stress. Mental stress is stress produced from reading, doing income taxes or balancing a bank book— stress caused by using the mind as a functioning element. Emotional stress includes, of course, those things that affect the emotions, such as fear, jealousy, anger, revenge, resentment or worry. Something that triggers the emotions is different from that which is merely the use of the brain for mental work. Physical stress is, of course, obviously simply the overfunctioning of the muscular system of the body.[2]

While on the subject of these three types of stresses, I might mention that in therapy, if a patient has a choice of exchanging one stress for the other, he should attempt to exchange them in a reverse order from which they are listed here. In other words, if it is possible to exchange an emotional stress for a mental stress, he should go ahead and do it since he will gain from the exchange. If he can exchange an emotional stress for a physical stress, this is even a better exchange. An example of such an exchange would be a patient who loves to go dancing but who overextends himself and exhausts his adrenal glands by his activities on the dance floor. However, he may be looking forward to a special dance so much that if he did not go, an emotional stress would be created that would probably outweigh the physical stress he will experience by going. In this instance, it is wiser for him to go to the dance and exchange an emotional stress for a physical one.

This same circumstance is often true regarding patients

---

[2] In our definition of physical stresses for this chapter we are referring only to those things the patient does as far as work and exercise are concerned. Certainly one could include such things as smoking, overeating, sleep deprivation, infection, pollution, temperature extremes, etc., as physical stresses but these are dealt with elsewhere in this text and are not a part of our thrust in this chapter.

and their employment, particularly married male patients. The physical and mental stresses involved in a CFS patient's work often tend to slow his recovery. However, his sense of family responsibilities and the nature of his individual character may be such that were he prevented from working, the emotional stresses of not being productive and being financially depressed may be far greater than the physical and the mental damage he creates by working. In these and similar instances, it is better to substitute one of the less injurious stresses for one more injurious.[3]

This same rule applies to exercise and the CFS patient. In fact, one of the most common questions I am asked by CFS patients is: "How much exercise should I take?" For the CFS patient, exercise must be considered as a physical stress and treated accordingly. This does not mean it should not be attempted—after all, physical stress is the least of the stresses—only that the patient must take certain precautions in its use. The master rule is: *As long as you feel no weakness or exhaustion the day following the exercise, you are all right and have not overdone. On the other hand, if you do feel exhaustion in the hours or days following the exercise, you have done too much.* The patient who has overdone must learn to reduce future exercise programs until he no longer experiences this exhaustion. In this manner, each CFS patient can find the optimal amount of exercise which is best suited to him.

---

[3] While proofreading this section, one of my editors left me this note: "Does this mean it's OK to eat junk food for emotional comfort? Or to fail to exercise because it's more agreeable to watch TV?" The answer to her question is not all that black and white. Much depends on the circumstances of the situation. The basic law of CFS regeneration is, "Do that which will create the least stress to the patient under the circumstances at the moment." Sometimes (but not often) this could mean a "Big Mac" is better than a "Big Mac attack." More often it does mean that it is better to sit and watch TV than do exercises that might act as an unneeded stimulant to a weakened adrenal gland. What is too much for a patient and what is allowable is to be determined by his physician from his long experience. It is for this reason that the efforts of a knowledgable doctor are essential for the management of the Chronic Fatigue Syndrome patient.

As the patient improves and neurohormonal tone is gained, the amount of exercise can be gradually increased. The amount of allowable increase must once again be ascertained by the procedure outlined above.

Proper exercise is an important part of the regime of the CFS in the Counterattack and Resistance Phases. Here the cortisol levels are high and carefully monitored exercise, along with the use of the phosphorylated mixture of L-Serine and Ethanolamine, are the main therapies used to moderate these elevated levels and give these patients some needed peace and rest.

The Rule of the Hand

Before we leave this subject, we should mention one of the most important, yet simple, techniques used to regulate the activities and exercise of the CFS patient. This is what I like to call, "The Rule of the Hand." It is important for every CFS patient to not use up his small amount of energy as he has in the past, or as the "normal" person does. Most of us, when we have a job to do, take it on and stay with it until it is finished. This determination and stick-to-itiveness is programed into us from childhood. While it is a worthy concept for the most of us, it is destructive to the CFS patient. When they attempt this procedure, they work until their adrenal gland is completely exhausted and forces them to stop. By the time they are forced to stop they have not only used up the energy generated by their treatments for regeneration of the adrenal gland but have actually weakened the gland further by attempting to force it to function beyond its abilities. It is efforts such as this that caused the CFS in the first place, and unless this practice is replaced with a more productive one, regeneration of the adrenal gland is not possible.

Their salvation is the Rule of the Hand and this rule is applied in this fashion. The patient is requested to look at the palm of their hand with the fingers extended. The fingers represent work or exercise periods, the web spaces between the fingers represent rest periods. Patients are admonished to use the Rule of the Hand to regulate their day. First they work or exercise for the few minutes (ten to twenty minutes depending on the degree of CFS the patient has) and then they rest for an equal time. Then they are allowed to do some work or exercise again for the same limited amount; this again to be followed by a rest period. This procedure is used throughout the day. At the end of the day the patients will find that they accomplished much more than they did previously but that the adrenal gland is much less stressed than previously, since it was allowed to regenerate during the frequent rest periods.

Obviously this method works best under the control of a physician knowledgable in the proper treatment of CFS. He must set the timing of the various intervals. This is vital to the success of this procedure. In the beginning for some patients the work (finger) periods must be very short and the rest (web space) periods long. As the patient improves, these are changed accordingly.

The Power of the Truth

In counseling for life-style stress reduction, one must remember that each patient is an individual problem (here the *"all are the same, all are different"* rule applies),[4] although some basic rules apply. It is important to build true rapport between the clinician and the patient. To this end, nothing is so powerful as the truth. I make it an unbreakable rule never to lie even in the slightest detail to a CFS patient. This penchant for truth is best engendered by the clinician's ardent desire to help his patient. More than this, the clinician has to learn to like his patient. If he cannot, it is probably wisest to refer the patient to another doctor. To become a CFS patient's healer, a clinician must become his friend. Almost no one else understands these patients. They are in a small lonely boat floating

---

[4] In my original work on this subject I coined this phase. It means this: All CFS patients follow the progression of the Selye chart and therefore are all the same, but since the symptoms of this condition are affected by the nature and heredity of each individual patient, they are all different.

in a sea of disbelief. The healer must constantly let them know that he understands their situation and that he is not only willing to help them, but he has the skill, knowledge and ability to do so. They require constant reassurance of the fact that they are going to get well, and to give them this reassurance the clinician must have the knowledge to get them well. Unless he can know in his own heart that he can get them well, his words will not be effective. People who are ill, and particularly individuals with CFS, are quick to pick up any sign of indifference or insincerity on the part of their practitioners.

Once a professional has earned the confidence of the CFS patient, he can begin to dissect and treat the patient's various stresses one by one. Sometimes, due to certain circumstances, major stresses cannot be approached at the beginning. Certain stresses may be too fearful for the patient to face or be of such a nature that the patient cannot yet accept their true character. The wise doctor will not become discouraged if the patient's response is slow at first. He may need to start with small treatable stresses. As these little stresses are worked out and the patient gains more confidence in him, the time will come when together the clinician and the patient can confront the larger stresses. This process is made much easier as the rest of the therapeutic regime strengthens the patient's adaptive mechanism.

I always think of each CFS patient as a beautiful jewel covered by a pile of debris. Each stress I help to remove is more garbage pulled off the pile. Eventually, I know, I will get to the jewel. Some pieces of garbage are small and some are large, but they all have to come off. Each one removed, no matter how small, moves me closer to the beauty of the jewel which I know is there.

Another general rule I use in this type of counseling is always to go forward, never back. I do not know how many times in my professional life I have quoted the biblical statement, "Let the dead bury the dead." That which has happened is done and gone; you cannot change it. The only thing that you can do is to go forward by obeying another biblical command, "what is that to thee? follow thou me."—*John* 21:22. Many chronic CFS patients have never really known a normal existence. They must build a new life, but to help them do this work, we must always proceed forward. This is the main thrust of our new Life Mastery course. This is a course of study especially designed to help the CFS patient go forward by becoming the Master of his life instead of its servant.

Group Therapy

In many instances, CFS patients seem to benefit from association with other patients with the same condition. In many of our programs, we utilize a form of group therapy to help them in their recovery. Unfortunately, it is possible to create harm if such group therapy is mishandled; therefore much care must be taken with this format. The physician must understand the various mechanisms involved, and each patient must evaluate the effect of such a group on his own nature before entering into a situation from which he cannot rapidly extricate himself.

One of the most common problems of the CFS patient is the loneliness he feels. It seems to him that all his friends are normal, and that he alone has this problem which no one he knows seems to understand or appreciate. Also, not having anyone with whom to compare notes, the patient cannot gauge the extent of his recovery or see evidence of anyone's recovering. The CFS patient is like a person at the bottom of a deep well. All he sees above him is a small, round shaft of light. His physician can tell him that there is a whole world of flowers, sunshine and beauty out there once he climbs to the top of the well, but it is hard for him to believe this while he is still stuck at the bottom of the well. To have the opportunity to talk with another patient who has successfully climbed out of the well and emerged into the sunshine can be a great boost to a struggling CFS patient. In this way the patient has someone who can understand his feelings and who can reassure him by example. An important part of the cure is often accomplished by the camaraderie that can be established among CFS patients.

The main precaution in using this "buddy" therapy is to prevent a weak patient from attaching himself to a stronger patient like a leech, expecting the stronger patient to help him through every little difficulty in his own life. Such practice can place an unfair stress on the stronger patient and lead to retrogression in his own condition. The wise clinician constantly watches that one of his CFS patients does not attempt to grow stronger by leeching strength from another.

The wise and alert physician also watches for conflicting personalities among his patients. Sometimes two patients are at the same stage of this condition, and therefore have a certain empathy for one another. Yet, by nature their personalities may be so different that one actually preys upon the other. In this situation it would be unwise for their physician to suggest that they attempt to help one another. When one directs an inpatient care facility, as we do at the Clymer Healing Research Center, one must keep an eternal vigil for destructive interplay between patients.

The nature of many CFS patients makes them sacrificing, helpful individuals. It is usually this sacrificing nature which produces many of the stresses which brought about their condition in the first place. Such a patient must be taught to respect his own needs and health care first. If he will not or cannot do this, he will not have the strength and energy necessary to help others. In these circumstances, little is gained by sacrificing one's own strength in an attempt to aid another person. It is the responsibility of every CFS patient to build his own individual strength before attempting to help others. Unless the patient is willing to do this, he will never find his own permanent recovery or cure.

Clinical Integration

The steps outlined above constitute the general clinical counseling program for CFS patients. One aspect of the program, however, has not been addressed. All parts must be integrated into a whole and, particularly in severe cases, presented to the patient in a controlled clinical environment. We do this by bringing patients into our Center for shorter or longer periods of composite treatment. Most patients with severe cases stay at our inpatient facility for a week or two to set up the necessary procedures and to begin preliminary counseling. If the case is not too severe, patients may then continue the proper therapy on an outpatient basis. The more severe cases may need to stay with us for extended periods, often one to three months. During this time, we are able to provide total commitment care, in which we control the entertainment they see, the food they eat, the air they breathe and the water they drink. In severe chronic CFS patients, only this total patient care is adequate to give improvement. Such patient care must not only be total, but individual. For example, CFS patients who suffer stress just waiting for their treatments are allowed to remain in their rooms until their treatments are ready so that they may rest as much as possible. Such measures, I am sure, seem extreme, but they are absolutely essential in severe CFS patients. However, with dedicated diligence and persistence even these patients may once again be returned to normal, healthy functioning.

One Step at a Time

As Benjamin Franklin wrote in his *Autobiography*, there was a time when he decided to correct all his bad habits. However, try as he would, he found it almost impossible to be good all of the time. He discovered that he could not concentrate on more than one bad habit at a time. Using these principles, he evolved a technique in which he wrote down all his bad habits and for a two-week period concentrated his entire being on one of his habits attempting to eliminate it. His presumption was that having worked hard on the habit for a fortnight, a certain residual effect would be produced in his system so that as he tackled each new habit, some of the good gained in fighting the previous habit would remain. Franklin repeated this procedure until, as he later stated, he was able to control all of his habits except that of pride. He assumed that even if he was finally able to overcome pride, he would be too proud of his accomplishment to call it a real elimination.

We have found a similar technique most effective in working with the stresses of the CFS patient. By taking one stress at a time, a patient can frequently conquer long-term stresses where only failure met him previously.

I am reminded of a recent patient who had a bad smoking habit, drank ten cups of coffee a day and had been on Valium® for many years. Any one of these habits would have been sufficient to prevent the progress of her condition, but all three made improvement nearly impossible. All attempts to help her by former physicians had failed. By following Franklin's method, we were able to work her off coffee first, then cigarettes and lastly the Valium.® Handling her in this manner, we were able to eliminate these noxious habits and finally treat and cure the CFS itself.

Many patients who come to us have suffered from CFS for many years. When they discover the length of time necessary for recovery, they often become discouraged. If they are willing to take their stresses one by one and work to correct them, they will see improvement in their entire being within a relatively short time. As they start to see these changes, they will develop enthusiasm for becoming an individual whose potential they had previously only imagined. According to a Chinese proverb, "A journey of a thousand miles starts with a single step." So it is with the stresses of the CFS patient. We must take them one by one; work on one and improve it before we go on to the next. No one can conquer all of the stresses in his life at once. We are after all only human beings, but as humans, we have free will and the possibility of an indomitable courage that will hold us in good stead as we work toward overcoming the various stresses that assault our bodies, minds and souls.

Summary

Therapeutic counseling, like the other treatment techniques, must be individually oriented and is one of the most important aspects of our treatment regime. Throughout the patient's entire program of regaining health and stability he must be willing to work with the doctor to overcome the various stresses in his life. This effort may need to be one stress at a time, but eventually all with be overcome.

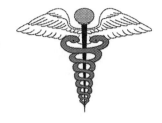

Chapter Nine

Nutritional Imbalances and Deficiencies

HE concept of nutritional imbalances and deficiencies is often debated in the treatment of CFS, as it is in the treatment and prevention of most conditions in the whole kaleidoscope of modern medicine. On one hand, there are physicians who contend that nutritional imbalances and deficiencies are the cause of nearly every disease known to mankind. On the other hand, there is that phalanx of medical orthodoxy that holds that except for a few rare diseases usually present only in other countries, such nutritional imbalances or deficiencies play little part in modern medicine. This disparity is somewhat similar to the controversy on hypoglycemia in that we feel the truth lies somewhere between the two extremes. One cannot help but wonder who in the long run does the greatest disservice to the honest promulgation of nutritional information—those who oversell this component of medicine or those who blatantly disregard it.

Importance of Therapeutic Balance

The correction of deficiencies and the establishment of a proper nutritional balance in the blood and tissues of CFS patients is absolutely essential to their recovery. Unless this is accomplished, all other treatment work can be much prolonged, and in certain instances thwarted entirely. However, four decades of experience in treating CFS has taught me that proper ingestion and absorption of the nutritional elements necessary to build the general adaptive mechanism are not in themselves sufficient to correct this syndrome.

The analogy I use to illustrate this conclusion to CFS patients is that of building a house. Proper nutritional needs of a patient are analogous to the materials necessary for proper house construction. Lumber, cement blocks, mortar, electrical wiring, plumbing supplies and roofing material are equivalent to the food we eat.

In the body as in the house, several considerations enter into the selection of the building material. We must know what kind of a house we are building. Is it a Spanish ranch house, a stone Victorian mansion or perhaps a Colonial saltbox? Obviously, the type of materials we select depends on the nature of the house. Each person's body is as different as these houses. Just as we would not order great amounts of brick and stone to build a Colonial saltbox, so we must be careful which specific nutrients we recommend for the CFS patient.

A builder, in choosing the materials for his house, orders the finest he can afford, those which are going to build a solid, enduring structure. To do less would be false economy indeed, for his house would no sooner be built than it would start to fall apart. This same situation applies to adrenal patients. Even though we may supply the proper foods, if the quality of those foods is poor, we will produce inferior results.

When building materials are to be ordered for the house, the builder must determine the intended size of the structure and decide how much of each type of material must be procured so that all the materials needed will be on hand with little or no waste incurred. The wise contractor spends a great deal of time considering the size and building specifications for any house he is about to build. In the same manner, a good clinician must give careful consideration to the treatment and management of his patient. Theoretically, the clinician should be even more thoughtful because a house is only a house, but a person is a human being—a temple of the living God.

Making Correct Choices

How does the clinician make the correct choices? On what does he base his opinion? Using the analogy of the house, one may ask, how do we know what kind of house we are building? How do we know which are the best materials? How do we know how much of each particular material to order?

The answer must start with the home-builder. He must conceive an idea of the type of house he wants; then he must consult with various architects until he finds one who will produce plans that properly depict his conception. Next a contractor must be commissioned who will carry out the plans in the manner conceived by the home-builder and depicted by the architect. At this time the proper materials may be selected and the construction of the structure begun. So it is with the treatment of the CFS patient, who in the analogy is the home-builder.

First, the patient must want to improve his situation—he must have the desire to make the effort necessary to regain his health, to build himself a new, more glorious "home." The effort should start with the search for the proper physician. This doctor will represent both architect and contractor to the patient. Working with the physician, the CFS patient must rebuild his neurohormonal system.

As a first step, the body must be thoroughly analyzed so that the proper nutritional needs can be determined. This chapter is devoted to explaining new and exciting methods for determining these nutritional needs. Before we delve into this subject, I wish to return to the house analogy for clarification of an important point. Supplying only the proper foods and nutritional supplements without the various regenerative treatments is the same as merely placing the materials on the building lot. These acts alone will not build the house, nor cure the CFS patient. Merely supplying the materials to build the house without actually hiring carpenters, plumbers, masons, electricians and so on is the same as supplying the nutritional elements to overcome CFS without utilizing the Magnatherm,

Myoflex, tissue sludge therapy, chiropractic adjustment, counseling facilities and all the other components that are necessary to rebuild strength and vitality in the patient's neurohormonal system. Many patients expect to overcome CFS by the use of nutritional substances alone. This concept is a fallacy. It is as insupportable as expecting to build a house by the mere acquisition and deposition of the necessary materials.

Accordingly, just as the construction of a house requires materials, workmen, a contractor and an architect to oversee the work, so must the CFS patient have a doctor who carefully balances each part of the patient's therapy so that recovery not only becomes possible but inevitable.

Modern Nutritional Analysis

As a whole, it is much easier for the contractor to supply the proper construction materials than it is for the clinician to determine and prescribe foods and supplements for the CFS patient. The doctor must ascertain the nutritional and chemical deficiencies and imbalances of the patient, know which substances will provide the optimal environment for correction and how much of each of the remedies the patient will require. These answers are not easily found. Fortunately, with the advance of computer technology and other improvements in laboratory equipment, we are now capable of analyzing the patient's tissues to discover levels of the elements in the body, and with this information determine what substances are needed to correct the deficiencies and imbalances.

Before I describe these new methods and techniques in detail, I wish to comment on past and present methods used by many nutritionists. In the beginning of medicine, little was understood about nutritional deficiencies and imbalances. As civilization and medical science advanced, knowledge of this subject began to evolve. Almost invariably, nutritional needs were discovered by the empirical correction of a symptom pattern or disease that had been unresponsive to previous treatment—such as the use of limes by the English sailors to overcome scurvy, rice polishings to counteract beriberi, or niacin-rich foods to cure pellagra. Soon nutritional elements were considered to be on a par with drugs and other medicinal compounds; they were used as a specific medicine to overcome a symptom or disease. We now know that many nutritional elements are needed by the body, and that if the body is to function properly, these must be available and *balanced*. To take vitamins and minerals indiscriminately without knowledge of the exact balance in a given case is to court trouble. To recommend one vitamin for one thing and another for something else is to ignore the need for a balance of vitamins and minerals in the body, for if any one vitamin is taken in greater than normal amounts for any length of time, it can create relative deficiencies of other nutrients.

The great early health advocates, such as Adelle Davis, Victor Lindlahr (the son of Henry Lindlahr, the author of our book *Nature Cure 2000*), and J. I. Rodale, recommended one substance for one condition, a second for another ailment, and so on. While all of these recommendations were made in good faith and undoubtedly achieved positive results, this method of prescribing nutritional supplements presents problems. It is difficult for a patient to assess a symptom pattern and reach a diagnosis. For instance, a patient may read that a certain element has given good results in the treatment of arthritis. What has proven helpful for one type of arthritis is not necessarily good for another, and such experimental treatment may actually exacerbate or aggravate his condition. He does know that he experiences aches and pains and that the remedy recommended by the health specialist sounds as if it might help. Perhaps the recommendation will help, perhaps not. It might push the system out of balance even more. Following this practice is akin to walking into a drugstore and asking the pharmacist for a prescription to alleviate a painful symptom. The pharmacist should recommend that the customer consult a physician to diagnose and treat the condition properly. Were the pharmacist to say, "Sure, try this. This helped Sally Jones, who had a pain in the same area a few weeks ago," he would definitely be out of line. This analogy is no more ridiculous than taking nutritional substances that purportedly aided someone else with similar complaints.

Indications and contraindications for use of nutritional substances in the treatment of disorders are just as specific as the indications for the use of drugs or other medications. Admittedly, most nutritional preparations are not harmful when used in small amounts. But when nutritional substances are used in large amounts such as are usually prescribed for therapeutic purposes, results can be disastrous if not used wisely.

While the pioneering work of the early nutritionists is laudable, attempting to apply their recommendations to health problems without first having the body mechanism thoroughly analyzed to ascertain actual needs or deficiencies does their memory and one's self a distinct disservice. Most lay people are not only prone to take the wrong element for the treatment of a condition, but they have no real idea of their own body's requirements. For example, if ten patients from our Center who had been diagnosed as having osteoarthritis were examined thoroughly for nutritional imbalances and deficiencies, almost invariably each would have needs different from the other nine. Therefore, a different nutritional program would be required for the proper correction of each disease state. Not only has a patient a disease, but a disease exists within a patient. The heredity and environment of each patient is different, and these differences produce a distinct set of nutritional imbalances and deficiencies. Unless these individual imbalances and deficiencies are ascertained and remedied, there is no real chance of long-term correction of the difficulty. The validity of this last statement would not be disputed by any reputable nutritionist or clinician, nor would it be opposed by any of the nutrition pioneers I have mentioned. The reason for the apparent conflict is that at the time these nutritionists reported their observations such methods of chemical analysis were not available, and therefore it was necessary for them to make general recommendations. I am sure they wholeheartedly believed it was better to give such recommendations than to omit the subject. I firmly believe that such decisions on their parts were correct at the time.

In any science or art, alert practitioners use the most advanced methods and techniques available to them. That is not to say that they do not wish they had superior methods available, but to wait until such methods are obtainable before imparting to humanity the work and understanding they have would be a great disservice. I shall presently outline advanced techniques for analyzing the nutritional needs of the human body. I am sure that ten years from now these state-of-the-art methods will be considered archaic. Undoubtedly, I will look back on this chapter and smile to myself at the methods suggested, but at this moment they are the finest and the most advanced methods known for nutritional analysis of the human body. What's more, they are effective; they give us information that has not been heretofore available and they help physicians cure their patients—which is, as they say in the oft-used cliche, "the bottom line."

Body/Nutritional Analysis

We use a set of tests known as the Chronic Fatigue Nutritional Profile at our Healing Research Centers. This nutritional analysis, originally developed at the Clymer Health Clinic, consists of an extensive blood-testing program (we were among the first to use, as a routine part of our blood-screening tests, lipoprotein electrophoresis, to measure fat levels; T-4 [Total Thyroxin], for thyroid function; ASO [Antistreptolysin 0] titer, to monitor or check for an infective condition; and RA [Rheumatoid factor] latex, to test susceptibility to rheumatoid arthritis); a tissue test for twenty-one minerals (toxic and nontoxic); a blood test for the twelve most common vitamins; a comprehensive diet analysis; hair analysis and a complete urinalysis.

The Chronic Fatigue Nutritional Profile is an exceptionally good diagnostic tool that has allowed us to recommend thousands of nutritional programs designed for the needs of the individual CFS patient. From the results of these test procedures, we are able to ascertain what substances an individual patient requires and the amount needed of each to balance the system. The experience of analyzing thousands of Chronic Fatigue Nutritional Profiles over many years has enabled us to ascertain which nutritional compounds are better absorbed and utilized and which are of lower quality and therefore are not recommended by our Centers.

The science of producing nutritional compounds is still in its infancy. For example, according to ingredients listed on the labels, several supplement products may seem similar, but in practice some combinations are much more effective than others. In addition, benefits derived from nutritional products vary from patient to patient. For instance, one adrenal substance may help twenty-four out of twenty-five patients, but cause one patient stomach discomfort or fail to bring about the desired improvement. For this patient, changing to another brand often corrects the problem. For these reasons we advise our patients to supplement only with the products we know are of value and can therefore recommend. The most important commodity the patient purchases from the physician is counsel and advice; not to consider and/or act upon the advice given is akin to throwing money away.

To make full use of the program it is essential that patients be retested every six months until such time that their body's chemistries are balanced. Thereafter, we recommend retesting once a year for maintenance purposes. By this protocol, we are able to analyze the best approach for handling individual problems, and also the most useful methods of correcting recurring problems.

Because this analysis program has revealed certain repeating groups of nutritional deficiencies, we can often diagnose a patient's difficulties from the pattern of the Chronic Fatigue Nutritional Profile. For instance, there is a Profile pattern for hypoglycemia, one for each of the various types of diabetes, one for many of the enigmatic mental disorders, as well as one for complications of CFS.

In the early days of my work I diagnosed CFS mainly from

changes in the postural blood pressure and from patient symptomatology. However, now we have discovered a specific pattern of nutritional imbalances in CFS patients, and whenever this imbalance manifests, we can, in my opinion, make a definitive diagnosis of CFS. This, of course, in conjunction with the definitive Adrenal Stress Index, since it is the ASI test that really allows us to determine the actual status of the CFS patient.

Occasionally we run into patients who, from all outward symptoms appear to have CFS, but whose ASI and nutritional analysis do not follow the usual patterns. Almost invariably, further examination of these patients shows that some other condition is causing the chronic debilitation. Both these tests have been of inestimable value to us, for they have saved our time and saved our patients from disappointment by allowing us to rapidly find, in most instances, the true causes of their symptom patterns.

Since our pioneering work with the Chronic Fatigue Nutritional Profile, other doctors and clinics are utilizing similar methods of patient analysis. As a humanitarian I must applaud this development, but as a clinician I must add a word of caution. The true benefit of the Chronic Fatigue Nutritional Profile comes not so much from the test procedure itself, but from the experience and skill of the clinicians who use the program. The technical methods involved in this type of program are delicate and complex, and from the clinical aspect it is easy to make mistakes unless the physicians involved are knowledgeable regarding CFS and highly motivated.

A Word of Caution

Frequently, companies that offer laboratory services attempt to persuade us to change to their company, assuring us that they offer advantages over services offered by the firms we now patronize. We carefully test the quality of services of each prospective laboratory by subjecting them to various tests designed to determine the effectiveness and accuracy of their methods. With laboratories who do hair testing, for instance, we take the hair of one individual, usually a member of our staff, divide it into two or three equal parts, and after it has been well mixed, send it on different days to one of the new companies, using assumed names. Ideally, all of the tests should report back similarly, because they are all portions of the same sample. In the companies we use regularly, the tests do provide nearly identical reports well within the accepted percentage of lab error. On the other hand, the sample readings from many of the competitive companies we have tested, even those of seemingly good repute, have come back so entirely different that we have judged their technology valueless.

In extreme instances we feel that our patients might even be injured if they followed the recommendations of these facilities, since it would be easily possible to increase certain deficiencies and exacerbate imbalances if a clinician used the hair or tissue analysis tests of these companies as a basis for his judgments. We always inform the subject companies of the results of our test studies after we receive their analyses in the hope that they might improve in the future. In one particularly flagrant case, a hair test laboratory rebutted by telling of all the other doctors who were satisfied with their work, but giving not a word of explanation as to why their reports on the same hair varied so greatly. We follow the same procedures with the laboratories that do blood testing and other analyses.

Admittedly, we are the bane of many nutritional testing companies. However, our patients' happiness and at times their very lives depend on the accuracy of our procedures, and we feel we must do all within our power to insure that these procedures are as accurate as is humanly possible.

Technology is now available for truly advanced nutritional testing; however, as this method of human analysis becomes better known, more "fly-by-night" outfits will be entering the field—firms that do not have the experience, skill or motivation to test accurately and whose procedures can possibly do more harm than good. A patient's best assurance is to seek a reputable clinic which will stand behind the results of its tests. Be especially careful of mail-order hair tests and those offered by health food stores. These sources have neither the knowledge nor the experience necessary to interpret or test the validity of their reports.

The Test Is Not the Answer

Results of nutritional testing that are obtained from these procedures must be looked upon in light of the patient's entire problem, and in light of the physician's experience with hundreds, or even thousands, of patients with similar difficulties and imbalances. This knowledge must then be combined with all the other findings to suggest the proper routine for each individual patient. It is not possible for a doctor who does a nutritional test now and then to understand the interplay and correlation of these results with the patient's other needs and requirements. One cannot simply take a tissue analysis test and, finding this mineral high and that mineral low, correct the problem by withdrawing the mineral that is high or supplying the mineral that is low. A mineral may be high or low in a test for many reasons. The mineral may be high not because the body has too much of it, but because the body is not able to utilize it properly, and therefore it is being stored in the hair or other tested tissues. Although the mineral appears high on a test, it may be one that is desperately needed by the body, but which must be supplied in a readily metabolized form other than that which the body is now receiving.

The fact that a mineral is low in the hair analysis does not necessarily mean that the body does not have sufficient amounts of this mineral; frequently this is true, but not always. Due to some other imbalance, the hair follicle may not be able to pick up the mineral, so that its amount in the hair could be low but body levels normal. This is common in the case of sodium if potassium is deficient. Sodium and potassium always tend to balance one another, and if the tissues are short in potassium, this usually shows in the hair; but to keep the proper balance, the hair follicle will not pick up more than enough sodium to balance the potassium, and so the sodium level will look low when it really is not. For these reasons a hair test is only as good as the laboratory which runs it and the clinician who interprets it.

The value of the Chronic Fatigue Nutritional Profile as given at our Centers is not necessarily in the numbers that are stated in the returned tests, but in these numbers as judged by our previous knowledge and in comparison with thousands of tests which have been taken previously. The information supplied by the Chronic Fatigue Nutritional Profile is not the "Word of God." It is simply important information that the doctor must utilize in his nutritional, supplemental, and dietary recommendations. His knowledge and experience, more than anything else, is the most vital part of the nutritional analysis.

Complete Mineral-Testing Procedure

As advanced and useful as the currently used Chronic Fatigue Nutritional Profile has been, I have long realized that for the best possible analysis of the nutritional states of our patients something further is required. As previously mentioned, a nutritional component may be high or low in the hair without showing the same fluctuation in the rest of the body. Heretofore, the analysis of the other bodily substances was not technically feasible because of the small amounts of minerals present and therefore the large amount of sample required to make an accurate testing. However, as a result of our constant requests, some of the more responsible tissue analysis firms have finally been able to develop a protocol by which the entire progress of nutritional elements in the body can be followed.

As nutritional substances are utilized, they are first taken from the digestive tract into the blood; from the blood they go to the various tissue repositories where they may be needed for body maintenance and repair; and, finally, those in excess or no longer of value are excreted in the urine. To have a truly accurate and complete analysis of nutritional elements in the body, we should know the state of these elements in the transporting mechanism (the blood), the accumulation of these minerals in the target or tissue elements (hair or finger-nails), and which elements and in what quantities are being excreted in the urine. Such a complex analysis is now available. While the cost of the complete mineral-testing procedure is somewhat higher than the Chronic Fatigue Nutritional Pro-file, it has been kept reasonable so that all persons who are truly interested in the needs of their body's nutritional health can avail themselves of this latest in advanced technology.

With the initiation of this complete mineral-testing pro-cedure, many of the honest objections that were raised regard-ing the hair analysis test have been overcome. Since we now analyze three different parameters of nutritional functioning in the body, our knowledge of this functioning has increased manyfold.

For example, if a certain mineral is normal in the blood, low in the hair, and high in the urine, we can readily assume that a sufficient amount is being taken into the body (because of the normal blood levels), but it is not being absorbed and metabolized by the body correctly (due to the low tissue levels and the high excretion levels). Enough of the element is coming in, but the body is not holding on to it; it is being lost through the urine. We know then that we have to do one of two things: find a form of this element that the body can use more readily, or work to normalize the digestive system of the body so that it can properly break down that nutrient. Usually in clinical practice we attempt to work on both these factors.

In another example, if a mineral is in normal quantity in the blood, high in the hair, and extremely low in urinary excretions, we now know that sufficient amounts of this element are being taken into the system, but that through some defect in metabolism it is being retained in the system and not being properly eliminated. This is common, for instance, with copper. In patients with a certain metabolic defect—often seen in those with CFS—copper cannot be excreted and accumulates in the system. Dramatic changes in personality can occur in this type of individual, because such an elevated copper level can cause mental and emotional symptoms which may border on those of schizophrenia. This condition is treatable through a proper combination of zinc, manganese and rutin, although it takes some time for recovery from the mental symptoms.

If an element is slightly high in the blood, quite high in the tissues, and is being excreted in fairly large amounts in the urine, the answer is obvious—the patient is taking in far too much of this element and the intake level should be reduced. On the other hand, if an element is slightly low in the blood, quite low in the hair, and being excreted also at a lower than normal level, we know that there is a definite deficiency in intake of this mineral. In this instance we must supply this mineral to a patient in the best-absorbable form available.

This method of analysis is of great value. Undoubtedly, in years to come new and more comprehensive techniques will be developed to give greater knowledge of a patient's nutritional needs. However, this new testing procedure along with those we have performed for many years enables us to provide comprehensive and exact help to CFS patients in finding their nutritional imbalances and deficiencies. In the past, a lack of this knowledge has been a weak spot in the treatment of this condition; it should be no longer.

Of all the so-called scientific advances of modern medicine, nutritional analysis is one I believe can truly qualify as an honest and useful aid to humanity. The ancients emblazoned over their temples, "Man, Know Thyself." This is what we are attempting to do with our methods of treatment. Every day and in every way we are trying to get to know our patients' "selves" better, and with these new methods of nutritional analysis we are closer to complete knowledge than ever before.

Summary

The correction of nutritional imbalances and deficiencies is an essential part of our treatment of CFS. To this end, all elements and substances the patient needs are determined by the best modern methods and then supplied to the patient to aid in their regeneration. To fulfill these aims, the Chronic Fatigue Nutritional Profile, a complete analysis of the body's nutritional mechanism originally developed at the Clymer Health Clinic, is essential. In addition to this profile, a three-way analysis—blood, hair, and urine—of the nutritional state of the body is now available. By the use of this triple nutritional analysis, the clinician can easily pinpoint and differentiate imbalances, deficiencies and over- and underingestion—not only to indicate what the patient needs, but to know in what form it must be given to be properly utilized. Even the finest of all of these tests, however, are of no lasting value unless they are backed up by extensive clinical experience and knowledge in their use and application by the physician in attendance.

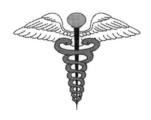

Chapter Ten

Stresses of the Environment—
Internal and External

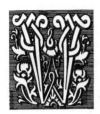HILE many of the stresses on the adrenal patient are obvious, others superimposed by environmental factors are not all that easy to ascertain. These stresses include those over which a patient exercises some control as well as those of an environmental nature that are mostly beyond his control. To release a patient from the grip of these stresses requires the physician's full skill and acumen. Those discussed here can be broken down into four groups:

1. Various chronic infective states that may be unrecognized.

2. Allergies—particularly to foods, pollen and toxic fumes.

3. Chemical toxicities—heavy metal and organic chemicals.

4. Miscellaneous stresses.

Many of these can be considered as diseases in and of themselves, but all of them may complicate a CFS case and therefore are germane to our subject.

Infective States

The direct connection between infective states and adrenal integrity has been well documented since the earliest research on this mechanism. Dr. Sajous' research contained many references to the adrenal glands and their relationship to infection.[1] This relationship may occur both as cause and as effect. It is often difficult to tell which came first—the weakened adrenal or the infection. Dr. Sajous stated that an adult with normally functioning adrenal glands is relatively resistant to all infections. On the other hand, my own experience and investigation have shown that infections place a heavy strain on the adrenal glands and can precipitate adrenal exhaustion, either temporarily, as in acute infections, or prolonged, as in the case of chronic infections. Therefore, whenever possible, the treatment of all infections should be directed to utilize the body's innate defense mechanisms, to strengthen and fortify these mechanisms and to prevent recurring infestations.

Probably the closest most people ever come to experiencing the symptoms of the adrenal exhaustion syndrome is during the period following an acute infection. Whenever an infective state triggers the fever-producing mechanism of the body, stress is placed on the adrenal gland system, since it is one of the main agents supplying the body with the energy it needs to be able to fight the infection. If the infection is severe or prolonged, the adrenal gland may become nearly exhausted by the time the infection is overcome. The weakness that frequently follows a case of influenza or a severe cold is merely an instance of exhausted adrenal glands demanding time and rest to regenerate themselves.

If the glands are permitted to rest and a person does not return to heavy activity (either mental or physical) until his full strength returns, the adrenal gland regains normal integrity and no permanent damage is done to the body's adaptive mechanism. However, if the patient returns to his daily duties before the adrenal gland is fully regenerated, there are several possibilities for damage to the adrenal gland, some more or less permanent. First, recovery may be much prolonged; the

---

[1] Sajous, Charles E. de M. *The Internal Secretions and the Practice of Medicine.* Philadelphia, F. A. Davis Company, 1903. (10th ed., 1922).

patient's adrenal glands may not fully recover their integrity for several weeks or even months following the infective ailment. Fortunately, most adrenal glands do eventually recover; however, much inefficiency and prolonged weakness could have been prevented if the individual had not attempted to return to his usual duties before his adrenal glands had had a proper time to recuperate following his infective condition.

In a second group of individuals, the gland regenerates to a functioning level, but does not rebuild completely to its previous state. The person with this condition is able to work and perform his duties as before, but the glands have been left weakened. This process may be repeated time after time with the adrenal gland becoming a little weaker after every bout of acute infection. Finally, the adrenal mechanism gives way due to the weakening created by the previous infections and the individual develops a full blown case of CFS. Our case history books are filled with records of such patients. Once this adrenal breakdown occurs, a person requires the same complex treatment as any other CFS patient.

In a third instance, we find some borderline adrenal insufficiency individuals who can be triggered into true CFS by only *one* severe acute infection in which proper regeneration of the adrenal gland is not allowed. Many of the CFS patients we see tell a story of how their condition began after a single case of flu or some similar acute infective condition.

Specific Infections

In addition to the general infections mentioned above, several specific types of infections are of great importance to the CFS patient. These fall into various categories.

First, the localized, acute infections. In this category are such complaints as boils, abscesses, streptococcal sore throat, pneumonia, cellulitis and phlebitis.

Second, acute systemic infections, both bacterial and viral. Here are such conditions as septicemia, childhood diseases (measles, chicken pox or mumps) and other acute systemic viral and bacterial infections.

Third, local, chronic infections, such as vaginal infections, fungus infections of the ear, *Candida albicans* infections of the vagina and herpes infections.

Fourth, chronic, systemic infections, a category which, it must be admitted, encroaches upon the third group, since most modern, research physicians believe that the basic infection in these instances is systemwide. Infections in this last category can be either of a severe or of a low-grade nature. In our work with the CFS patient, we are more interested in the low-grade chronic, systemic infections, since they are more likely to go undiagnosed and untreated.

Acute Local Infections

While acute local infections may have adverse effects on the adrenal mechanism, they are usually of a type that readily falls within the expertise of modern orthodox medicine, and today these infections only rarely are the cause of adrenal exhaustion leading to CFS. Improved sanitary conditions, the knowledge and use of nutritional compounds, particularly vitamin C, and the judicious use of antibiotics have helped mankind make great strides in overcoming these once-common causes of death. Most are of bacterial origin, and whenever they appear are usually well handled by antibiotic therapy.

In our Healing Research Centers, we use antibiotics only when other forms of more natural therapy have not been able to correct an infection. We attempt to stimulate the body's defense mechanism to overcome acute infections. In this technique, the defense mechanism gains strength by honing the process of antibody formation and directing its own forces. All this is accomplished in the same manner that a battalion of soldiers gain skill and wisdom in fighting by becoming seasoned in battle. When antibiotics are given, the body's mechanisms are not required to control the infection, and no true seasoning of this mechanism can occur. Thus, the body's own defense mechanism remains weak and the patient is inclined to "catch" every "bug" that is "going around."

In acute, local infections, whether treated by use of antibiotics or by the natural methods we prefer, the condition is usually quickly overcome and stress on the adrenal glands, though perhaps severe for a short time, is not prolonged and does not tend to cause permanent damage unless the patient does not allow sufficient recovery time after the infection has subsided. The postinfection recovery time required is similar to that described for the common cold or for flu.

The remarks concerning acute, local infective conditions also apply to the acute systemic variety, except for greater emphasis on both trying to let the body do as much of the work as it can and allowing sufficient time for adrenal recovery following the acute stage of the infection. This can take weeks or months in severe acute systemic infection. As mentioned previously, a good half of all our CFS patients can trace back the beginning of their condition to an infection of some sort from which they did not allow sufficient recovery time.[2]

Chronic Infective Conditions

In chronic infective conditions, the local manifestation often is only a coming to the surface of an internal systemic infection, and therefore both local and systemic chronic infections should be handled together.

In the treatment of recalcitrant CFS patients, the whole area of low-grade chronic infection is fertile soil for investigation. When the adrenal mechanism becomes lowered in efficiency, the body frequently loses its ability to control a group of parasitic organisms that usually abound on its surfaces and membranes. Studies with new electronic microscopes have found throughout the body almost every dangerous bacterium and virus known to man. Fortunately, most individuals have within them a symbiotic relationship that prevents these organisms from becoming injurious to their health. The resistance of the body—and when I say resistance I am speaking almost specifically of those mechanisms that are controlled by

---

[2] The control of acute infections is treated fully in our books *It's Only Natural* and *Nature Cure 2000*. We recommend these texts for those who desire more information on this aspect of natural healing.

the adrenal glands—prevents any adverse effects from these uninvited guests. However, as a person's resistance (the adrenal mechanism) becomes less competent, either temporarily or permanently, these parasites are no longer capable of being controlled, and various forms of infective flare-ups occur in the body. In many instances, all that is necessary to control these low-grade infections is the general support of the adrenal mechanism as discussed in this book. However, in the many instances in which the infection has achieved a toehold, this general support is not adequate, and specific measures must be taken to rid the body of the chronic infective condition.

In handling many of these chronic conditions, antibiotics have little or at best limited use. To understand this, it is necessary to have an understanding of the basic working of the antibiotic. Despite popular opinion, antibiotics do not, per se, kill bacteria. They only prevent them from reproducing. In acute infections, huge numbers of bacteria reproduce at such a rapid rate that their toxins could be fatal to the system if not reduced. The antibiotics are used to reduce the bacterial hordes to amounts that the body's defense mechanism can overcome. Once the level of bacteria is reduced to a certain point, the antibiotic effect is negligible, and only the body's own processes can eliminate the remaining survivors. In most chronic infections, the level of bacterial proliferation remains below that for which antibiotics are really effective. If antibiotics are given, the most they can do is to prevent acute exacerbations, but they are not usually able to correct the chronic infection itself. A typical case in point is the use of tetracycline to treat acne. This antibiotic can be used to prevent severe eruptions, but it does not eliminate the chronic infection. In low-grade chronic infections, the residual bacteria, though below the level which are affected by the antibiotics, are still sufficient to cause severe stresses on the adrenal mechanism.

Many chronic infections are of the viral or fungal variety such as the common herpes and the *Candida albicans* infections. Antibiotics have absolutely no effect on these organisms.

It would seem as if the discovery and use of wonder drugs has kept us from grave dangers of severe acute infections, only to leave us with a background of low-grade chronic infections which are debilitating to vast numbers of our population. This subject of low-grade chronic infection is one that will be investigated for many years to come. In my opinion, many of the present enigmatic chronic diseases for which medicine knows no cause or cure are actually unknown manifestations of known chronic infections, or low-grade chronic infestations of organisms yet to be discovered.

Among the important chronic infections which are understood and are treatable are conditions caused by *Candida albicans*, the various herpes viruses, Lyme disease spirochete and *Staphylococcus aureus*. But, we feel that these are only the tip of the iceberg and that there are a great many of what my colleague, Dr. Harold Buttram, calls "slow viruses" that are causing chronic stresses in many of our CFS patients. These viruses are difficult to eradicate or even to detect. Frequently, we have found that patients with a "slow virus" will run low-grade temperatures in the 99° to 100° range. These patients also seem warmer to the touch than the average patient even when they are not running a temperature.

We find many patients with such chronic viral infections respond well to our regular immune system enhancement treatments, but for others we need to utilize a variety of specialized state-of-the-art therapies to eradicate their unwanted guests. To this end we have such exotic treatments as blood transluminescense (some of a patient's blood is removed, irradiated with ultraviolet light to kill the offending organism and the blood then replaced in the body), Total Octazone[3] Absorption (The patient is placed in a large airtight bag with only the head free and the bag is filled with Octazone, a very reactive form of ozone. The Octazone is absorbed by the

---

[3] Octazone is a substance supposed to be composed of a molecule with eight atoms of oxygen. This may or may not be true, but it does work.

skin and acts to kill the slow viruses in the blood.), the use of the Rife technique to kill the chronic organisms by exposing them to vibratory frequencies that shatter their outer capsule, the use of special nontoxic substances to increase the activity of "killer" white cells in the blood, etc.

Several of these state-of-the-art treatments are still investigational and are not covered by most insurances. After all, according to the medical consensus, there is no known effective treatment for CFS, therefore all treatment that works must be considered "investigational." Since most of the work we do at our Clinics is for those patients that have been declared "incurable" by their regular physicians, we call ourselves Healing Research Centers. In other words, treatment by the "consensus of medical opinion" has failed our patients. Therefore, everything we do is unique, state-of-the-art and research in one form or another.

In our book *Adrenal Syndrome*, first published in 1983, we mentioned a disease agent called *Progenitor cryptocides*.[4-8] This was a bacterium discovered by Drs. Virginia Livingston Wheeler and Eleanor Alexander-Jackson. At that time Dr.

---

[4] Wuerthele-Caspe, Virginia, and others. Cultural properties and pathogenecity of certain microorganisms obtained from various proliferative and neoplastic diseases. *American Journal of Medical Science* 220:638-648, December 1950.

[5] Wuerthele-Caspe, Virginia, and others. Intracellular acid-fast microorganism. *Journal of American Medical Women's Association* 11(4):120-129, April 1956.

[6] Livingston, Virginia Wuerthele-Caspe, and Livingston, Afton Munck. Some cultural, immunological and biochemical properties of Progenitor cryptocides. *Transactions of the New York Academy of Science,* Series 1136(6):569-582, June 1974.

[7] Livingston, Virginia Wuerthele-Caspe, and Livingston, Afton Munk. Demonstration of Progenitor cryptocides in the blood of patients with collagen and neoplastic diseases. *Transactions of the New York Academy of Science* 34(5):433 453, 1972.

[8] Livingston, Virginia Wuerthele-Caspe, and Livingston, Afton Munk. A specific type of organism cultivated from malignancy: Bacteriology and proposed classification. *Annals of the New York Academy of Science* 174:636-654, October 30, 1970.

Alexander-Jackson was making a vaccine to be used to eliminate this organism. We had a great deal of success with this
vaccine in those patients who demonstrated the *Progenitor
cryptocides* in the living blood under the dark field microscope
(the only way it could be readily detected). However, since the
passing of both these pioneers, this vaccine is no longer
available and is greatly missed by us and our patients. We still
do the live blood cell examinations (with much improved
equipment over that used in 1983) and are now correlating
these results with our newer therapies mentioned above. Since
I see no reason to expect that the *Progenitor cryptocides* agent
has disappeared just because its discoverers have left this
planet for parts unknown, we have decided to include in this
work our original information on this subject. Who knows,
maybe some brilliant young researcher will read this and
decide to go on safari in the human body and once again track
down this wild beast, known as *Progenitor cryptocides*.

Progenitor cryptocides

One of the most fascinating research projects
concerning these low-grade chronic infections
is the work of Dr. Virginia Livingston Wheeler
and Dr. Eleanor AlexanderJackson. These two
have for many years worked on a little-known
bacterium called *Progenitor cryptocides*. Their
research has proven that this agent is present in
almost all human beings. Controlled in most
of us, it can cause a variety of disease patterns
in those who are susceptible. This organism,
Progenitor cryptocides, is unique in that it is
pleomorphic, that is, it has the ability to change
its shape and appearance under different circumstances. Therefore, these doctors believe
that it is the offending agent in many conditions for which other organisms have been
indicted.

This organism is also unique in that it can be observed in the living blood of patients if a proper type of dark-field examination is made. The degree of infestation and response to treatment can be easily and rapidly monitored by this method.

It is essential to be on the lookout for *Progenitor cryptocides* infection in all Adrenal Syndrome [CFS] patients. The discovery and correction of this type of infection can often make the difference between their improvement and their steady decline.

The patient's history usually reveals if he is infected with *Progenitor cryptocides*. Patients who demonstrate occasional low-grade fevers for which there is no specific known cause, who have unexplained joint aches and pains that resemble what once was called rheumatism, who have symptoms of fatigue and general lack of energy which do not seem to fit any known pattern, or in whom treatment has proven ineffective should be checked for possible infection with *Progenitor cryptocides*.

In our Clinic, all patients who come for a general examination are given the dark-field investigation of the living blood. If we find by this test a high percentage of cryptocide organisms, urine culture is made. If this is positive, the diagnosis is specific and an autogenous vaccine (one that is made from the patient's own bacteria) is ordered. Experience has shown that while it is essential to support the general adaptive mechanism in these cases, a real cure is not usually possible until the autogenous vaccine (developed and still produced by Drs. Livingston and Jackson) is utilized.

The use of the vaccine has proven a true godsend to a large number of our Clinic patients.
It has helped patients overcome many conditions that previously had resisted the best of
our work and orthodox medical practices.

Candida albicans

Among the most common chronic infections that afflict
the CFS patient today is the yeast infection *Candida albicans*.
Through the original work of C. Orian Truss, M.D., we have
become conscious of the fact that *Candida albicans* can become a systemic infection and affect not only women, but also
men.[9-11] It has, as described by Dr. Truss, the ability to cause a
variety of cerebral allergic reactions. It has been known to be
sufficiently severe to precipitate suicide. The functioning
mechanism is somewhat similar to that of *Progenitor cryptocides*
infections, in that the agent is, according to Dr. Truss, in nearly
100 percent of our population. In most, it is held in abeyance
by the body's defensive mechanism. If this mechanism becomes lax, as in the case of CFS, this agent easily becomes more
virulent and systemic. Doctors who have researched this agent
believe that since it is present in most vaginas, it is passed on
to children, both male and female, during the traverse of the
birth canal. Interestingly, symptom patterns which can be
produced by this agent closely mimic those of CFS itself and its
frequent companion, hypoglycemia. The cerebral allergies
produced by *candida*'s toxicants produce in some people
symptoms mimicking various mental derangements. *Candida albicans* infections can often be picked up from the
general history of the patient. Any female patient who has had

---

[9] Truss, C. Orian. Restoration of immunologic competence to *Candida
albicans*. *Journal of Orthomolecular Psychiatry* 9(4):287-301, 1980.

[10] Truss, C. Orian. Role of *Candida albicans* in human illness. *Journal of
Orthomolecular Psychiatry* 10(4):228, 198 1.

[11] Truss, C. Orian. Tissue injury induced by *Candida albicans*. *Journal of
Orthontolecular Psychiatry* 7(1):17-37, 1978.

a history of yeast infections and who demonstrates some of the bizarre symptoms mentioned above should be investigated for possible systemic *candida* infection.

In many cases, however, it is difficult to ascertain whether a *candida* infection is systemic. Perhaps the best differential diagnosis is one using the response to specific therapy. The oral agent used to control *candida* infections is an antifungal called Nystatin;[12] another trade name is Mycostatin®.[13] One might consider Mycostatin® or Nystatin an antibiotic for yeast substances. Fortunately, unlike the bacterial antibiotics, these antifungal drugs have a low incidence of side effects, due to the fact that there are, as far as we know, no beneficial yeasts in the body. Unlike antibiotics, that can prevent the reproduction of the beneficial bacteria in our body as well as the nonbeneficial, Mycostatin® and Nystatin affect only the detrimental yeasts. Furthermore, these agents are not absorbed in the system but stay in the digestive tract if ingested and in the vagina if inserted there. This explains their low toxicity.

If a patient is suspected of having systemic *Candida albicans* infection, a short schedule of Mycostatin® or Nystatin usually helps clear up many of the systemic symptoms. If this does occur, we can be safe in assuming that they were caused by the systemic *candida* because there are no other effects of the antifungal treatment. On the other hand, if the patient does not benefit from a course of Mycostatin® or Nystatin, it does not necessarily mean that that patient is not bothered with a systemic *candida* problem, as some patients do not respond to these drugs. In these cases, we use a specific *candida* vaccine similar to that used for the *Progenitor cryptocides*, except that this is a general vaccine and not an autogenous one, as in the case of *Progenitor cryptocides*. This vaccine, with or without the antifungal, has proved successful in most cases. Although much remains to be learned about yeast and fungus infections,

---

[12] Prepared by Lederle Laboratories, Division of American Cyanamid Company, One Cyanamid Plaza, Wayne, NJ 07470.

[13] Prepared by E. R. Squibb & Sons, Inc., General Offices, P.O. Box 4000, Princeton, NJ 08540.

recent research has focused on the blocking relationship between *candida* and hormones, showing how *candida* can impair their function.[14-15] As bodily hormones are secreted, they go by nature to a specific receptor site in a specific organ, similar to the way a key fits into a lock. With *candida* organisms, however, it is as if a counterfeit key, a hormone-like substance—such as an estrogen-like or an adrenocortical-like product—slips into the lock and blocks the reception of the body's own hormones by an organ. Normal hormonal function is impaired. Thus, *Candida albicans* is now recognized as one of the mechanisms by which CFS can be triggered. Now that a breakthrough has been made and *Candida albicans* is recognized as a source of possible chronic infection, it is hoped that more work will be done in this area.

Since the above was originally written, there has been a great deal of investigation into *Candida albicans* as it is accepted by the orthodox medical community. The systemic drug of choice today is Diflucan®.[16] This has replaced Nizoral®.[17] Both of these drugs, unlike Nystatin, do enter the blood and are therefore able to work on *Candida albicans* that has left the vagina or digestive system and become truly systemic. As a trade-off for this efficiency both of these drugs are much more toxic than the rather innocuous Nystatin.

Even with these new powerful drugs, however, we do not have the final answer to *Candida albicans*. These drugs act much like antibiotics in that they are able to reduce the population of the *Candida albicans* but are not able to cure the condition. Here again we need to attend to the immune system and the adrenal gland's contribution to its integrity.

---

[14] Loose, D. S., Schurman, D.J., and Feldman, David. *Nature* 293:477, 1981.

[15] Feldman, David, and others. An estrogen-binding protein and endogenous ligand in Saccharomyces cerevisial: Possible hormone receptor system. *Science* 218:297-298, October 15, 1982.

[16] Prepared by Roerig Division, Pfizer Incorporated, 235 East 42nd Street, New York, NY 10017.

[17] Prepared by Janssen Pharmaceutica, Inc., 40 Kingsbridge Rd., Piscataway, NJ 08855.

Without these factors, both antibiotics and antifungals give only temporary assistance in chronic infections.

There are a number of natural remedies to help the CFS patient with *Candida albicans* until the immune system can be regenerated. They are too numerous to discuss here, but if *Candida albicans* is one of your problems, be certain to mention it to your Healing Research Center physician.

The diet of the *Candida albicans* patient is vital to his recovery and such a diet is offered in Appendix I.

Genital Herpes

One of the most common prevailing low-grade infections at the present time is herpes virus II. There are, of course, various forms of the herpes virus, from the common mouth ulcer or canker sore, the lip lesion known as a cold sore, to that which forms the nerve infection of shingles. The most important to the CFS patient, however, is the venereal form, type II, which occurs on the genitalia of both male and female. There has been a tremendous increase in this latest form of herpes due to the increased promiscuity of our sexually liberated society. Those who have read my books *Creative Sex*[18] or *One Flesh*[19] are undoubtedly familiar with my thoughts on this subject; however, as a physician it is not my duty to moralize, but to do all I can to help my patients live more productive lives, whatever their own moral convictions or habits.

Herpes is a perfect example of that agent that is dependent on the weakness of the general adaptive mechanism of the body for its manifestation. People who have the low-grade systemic herpes II infection know all too well that it will show up if they eat the wrong types of foods, do not get sufficient rest, or abuse themselves physically or emotionally. It has been my experience that the condition of the herpes is more dependent on the state of the adrenal mechanism than the adrenal

---

[18] Poesnecker, G.E. *Creative Sex.* Quakertown, PA, Clymer Health Clinic, 1976.

[19] Poesnecker, G.E. *One Flesh.* Quakertown, PA, Humanitarian Publishing Company, 1996.

mechanism is dependent on the state of the herpes. Herpes, I find, is not a particularly disabling infection to the adrenal mechanism; however, by supporting the adrenal mechanism, patients who have this infection may be helped.

Experience has proven that the herbal remedies echinacea, myrrh and thuja—particularly thuja—can be effective in controlling this agent, assuming the patient is not otherwise dissipating, thereby causing undue strain on his adaptive mechanism. Sugar also seems to be a sensitizing compound to certain forms of the herpes virus. If a patient, particularly one afflicted with fever blisters or canker sores, consumes too much sugar and an insufficient amount of phosphorus-free calcium in the form of calcium carbonate, citrate or lactate, the mouth ulcers tend to manifest much more frequently.

Recently, research has shown that the amino acid lysine tends to counteract the herpes infection, and many authors are now recommending its use as a treatment for these chronic infections.[20-21]

Personally, it is against my principles to take one substance, even though it is a natural substance, out of its matrix and give it in larger than normal amounts to the body. I fear it may in turn create other imbalances which could eventually cause greater problems than the one for which it was prescribed. Time may prove me wrong on lysine, but maybe not.

Lyme Disease

When I wrote the first edition of this work, Lyme disease was just making the headlines. Nobody was very certain what caused it and so it was not included in that first edition entitled *Adrenal Syndrome*. We now must include Lyme disease since it is one of the most common chronic infections complicating CFS. At least this is true in the Northeastern part of our nation.

---

[20] Griffith, R. S., and others. Relation of arginine-lysine antagonism to herpes simplex growth in tissue culture. *Chemotherapy* 27(3):209- 213, 1981.

[21] Lysine prophylaxis in recurrent herpes simplex tabialis: A double-blind, controlled crossover study. *Acta Dermato-Venereologica* (Stockholm) 60(L):8587, 1980.

Lyme disease is caused by an agent known as *Borrelia*. This agent is spread to humans by a small deer tick. This tick is very hard to spot since it is much smaller than the usual dog tick that is so common in many parts of the country. The bite of this tick leaves a unique "bull's eye" marking around the area where the skin was broken. The early diagnosis can be made from this marking and from the early symptoms of pain in the muscles and joints. Antibiotics are the therapy of choice at this time, but while these are effective in treating the acute stage, they usually do not eliminate the agent, and if the adrenal gland–immune systems are compromised, the symptoms can return at a later date. If they are severe, antibiotics can be used to again reduce the agent population, but the symptoms will appear again and again if the adrenal gland-immune systems are not regenerated.

Chronic Staphylococcal Infections

The chronic infection *Staphylococcus aureus* is among the most ancient of all known human infections. Usually, this is the infective organism whenever pus is formed. The encouraging thing about staphylococcal infections is that they are generally circumscribed, that is, the body tends to wall them off so that they can be controlled. Because of this, they do not generally spread systemically. The agent may be systemic at times, but the manifestation is usually local and tends to work toward the surface whenever possible. Boils, carbuncles, abscesses, so-called "teen age pimples," and, of course, lesions of acne are all staphylococcal infections. While most of these infections are acute in nature and therefore do not have a prolonged effect on the CFS patient, they are certainly a stress and should be eliminated if at all possible.

Those staphylococcal infections that do become chronic present a real stress on any individual. These need to be tracked down and eliminated by the various natural therapies available to our Centers' physicians.

The staphylococcal germ has shown an ability to build up a resistance to various forms of antibiotics. In fact, several years ago we often heard the term, "Hospital Staph," which was the common name of a staphylococcal germ that had lived in the world of hospital antibiotics to such an extent that it built up an immunity to them. Since the heaviest use of antibiotics occurred in hospitals, this was where the germ lived. During this time, hospitals became some of the most dangerous places on earth to inhabit. As a result of better cleanliness and upgraded handling of various types of disease, this situation has been better controlled. However, the staph germ still is far from being conquered by modern orthodox medicine. The chronic, systemic form, as is present in cases such as acne, can be controlled by various antibiotics, but cannot be eliminated from the system by these drugs. We once had a very good remedy for this condition, but a few years ago the FDA did its usual magic trick and made it disappear from the market. The name of this product was staphage lysate.[22]

Staphage lysate was a bacteriophage culture that helped to stimulate the body's ability to build what are called macrophage or scavenger cells, which work to eliminate the chronic staphylococcal infection. Staphage lysate seemed to have no side effects and, for cases in which antibiotic therapy provided only temporary results, it often proved to provide a cure.

Allergies and CFS

It is necessary to diagnose and treat a CFS patient's specific allergy(ies), although such treatment, in the beginning, is only a stopgap mechanism until the patient's general adaptive system is built up. Only by establishing normal function in this system can the patient be kept truly resistant and free of these allergic sensitivities. Adrenal insufficiency causes allergies, and allergies weaken the adrenals. Therefore, to establish a cure, it is necessary to work from both ends toward the middle. The general adaptive mechanism must be built up to help control the allergies, and the allergies must be controlled to reduce the stress on the general adaptive mechanism.

---

[22] Originally produced by Delmont Laboratories, Inc., Box AA, Swarthmore, PA 19081.

Identifying Food and Other Fixed Allergies

For many years we have realized that many CFS patients have shown abnormal sensitivities to certain foods. Some of these allergic-like food problems can be detected and corrected by known diagnostic and therapeutic measures. Unfortunately, however, the great majority of them remain an enigma to us. In recent years, the technology for detecting various food sensitivities has advanced greatly. Our Woodlands Healing Research Center has devoted a great deal of time and energy to this part of the CFS treatment and is considered as one of the nation's leaders in this area.

Dr. John W. Tintera believed that all allergies and allergic reactions result from a weakening of the adrenal system.[23-24] If this is true, and I see little reason to doubt it, it is readily understood why so many CFS patients have frequent allergic reactions.

The CFS patient can be sensitive to many allergy-producing substances, of which food allergies are the most ignored and undetected. The food allergies with which most people are familiar are those known by doctors as fixed allergies, that is, a substance which always reacts with an individual patient whenever he comes in contact with this food, no matter how small the amount may be or how long it has been since he last encountered it. For instance, some patients break out whenever they eat tomatoes. The symptomatic reaction is of no great consequence in the diagnosis of the condition. It does not matter whether they get a stomachache, a rash or merely become dizzy, these are individual reactions to the allergic shock to the system from the ingestion of the food. Most people who have fixed allergies know all too well which substances cause their reactions, for the reactions are usually dramatic and sudden.

---

[23] Tintera, John W. The hypoadrenocortical state and its management. *New York State Journal of Medicine* 55:1869, 1955.

[24] Tintera, John W. What you should know about your glands and allergies. *Woman's Day* February 1959, pp. 28-29,92.

As a patient's general adaptive mechanism is supported and strengthened by the procedures discussed in this book, some of the fixed allergies may improve. However, most fixed allergies are well entrenched in the genetic structure of the patient, and it may not be possible to eliminate them in one lifetime. For comfort, he must stay away from the offending substance. Usually, fixed-food allergies are not a serious problem in the CFS patient, since forced abstinence prevents symptoms and therefore stress.

The number of fixed allergies is usually small compared with the number of cyclic allergies, which is the type commonly found in CFS patients. A variable or cyclic allergy is caused by the short-term buildup of antibodies in the system which are produced to react to a certain substance. They will abate within a few days if this food is not soon repeated. For example, if a person who has a cyclic allergy to milk and drinks milk every day, certain antibodies accumulate in the blood which eventually react with the milk metabolites also present in the blood. This reaction is usually not as severe as that of a fixed allergy, but is more insidious, often producing what are known as cerebral allergies—toxic substances which affect the brain and produce a mild stultifying effect on the whole body. This allergy may destroy the sense of well-being so cherished by us all. These antibodies will remain in the blood, and the reactions will continue to occur as long as the person drinks milk. However, if milk is withheld for four or five days, the antibodies in the blood will abate, for they have a short life span unless reinforced by continual ingestion of the allergic food. After a week, most antibodies will have left the blood, and so, although the person is still sensitive to milk, he could take a small amount without serious trouble. This is the mechanism behind the diet regimen necessary for controlling, and the testing procedure needed to detect, specific cyclic food allergies.

Actually, the cyclic allergy is not a true allergy, but a side effect of the body's attempt at self-protection. It occurs because a weakened digestive system does not break down food particles properly and incompletely digested particles enter the bloodstream. The protective mechanism of the blood reacts to them, as it would to any foreign object, by producing antibodies to rid the body of these substances.

The ideal treatment for this condition is one that enables the digestive system to break down foods completely, so they do not enter the bloodstream partially digested. Unfortunately, digestive weakness is one of the first products of CFS. Therefore, it is little wonder that these cyclic allergies are so common in CFS patients.

In treating the CFS patient, we must do everything we can to improve his digestive mechanism. In many instances, by the time we see a patient, the problem has been entrenched for many years, and the digestive mechanism is extremely poor. In fact, many patients can no longer digest and metabolize the nutritional substances which are essential to building the general adaptive mechanism. For these patients we must find and reduce the cyclic allergies before the digestion can be improved.

Much of the developmental work with this type of food-allergy testing was done by the psychiatrist Dr. William Henry Philpott, who worked out a four-day food-rotation diet which takes into consideration specific foods and also specific families of foods for which there might be some cross-sensitization in patients.[25-26] Our modification of this four-day rotation plan is included in Appendix 1. We find this plan of use to many patients, particularly since it gives information on the food families. Some patients are so sensitive that even though they stay away from a certain food, if they use a food of the same family, they may sustain antibody reactions. This plan need not be slavishly followed. It is presented only as an example of a diet that does allow a five-day hiatus between the

---

[25] Philpott, William Henry. Ecologic, orthomolecular and behavioral contributions to psychiatry. *Journal of Orthomolecular Psychiatry* 3(4):356-370, 1974. (See especially pp. 359-360.)

[26] Philpott, William Henry. Four-day rotation diet. *Clinical Ecology*, edited by Lawrence D. Dickey. Springfield, IL, Charles C Thomas, 1976.

use of certain food families and yet offers adequate nutrition and substance.

While this is a simple procedure and costs the patient nothing (except for the different types of foods), we do find it very effective for many CFS patients. The power of such simple changes was brought home to us early in our treatment of this condition by the beneficial results many of our patients had when they travelled abroad. At first when CFS patients told me that they were going to take a trip to Europe I was very concerned about their diet in a strange environment, but when almost all of them returned home feeling great and assuring me that the food agreed with them perfectly, I began to look for an answer. Soon it was obvious to me that since they were being exposed to foods and preparation that their body had never encountered before, it had no antibodies to react. So their trip was actually like a glorified rotation diet. This concept was given further verification by one patient who stayed in Europe for some time. After a few weeks she again began to experience the difficulty she had at home as her body was beginning to build antibodies to her new foods.

Provocative Testing

Sublingual and subcutaneous provocative testing, a method made popular by Dr. Marshall Mandell of Norwalk, Connecticut, consists of placing the patient in a contamination-free environment and putting extracts of various substances under the subject's tongue or injecting them into the arm.[27-28] The physician then watches for several minutes and notes specific reactions. If reactions occur, the doctor can use a homeopathic dilution of the same substance tested in an attempt to find a specific desensitizing dose. For example, if a patient is being tested for gasoline fumes, a certain extract

---

[27] Mandell, Marshall, *Cerebral Reactions in Allergic Patients.* Presented at the 24th Annual Congress, American College of Allergists, Section on Neurologic Allergy, Washington, DC, April 18, 1969.

[28] Mandell, Marshall, and Scanlon, L. W. *Dr. Mandell's 5-Day Allergy Relief System.* New York, Thomas Y. Crowell Co., 1979.

containing this substance is placed under the patient's tongue. After a few minutes, if the patient is sensitive to the substance, he starts to display a variety of symptomatic reactions, such as headache, dizziness, sleepiness, numbness, strange sensations in different parts of the body, or any one of the innumerable allergic type reactions. When these begin to occur, and if it is desired to desensitize the patient from the specific substance, different homeopathic dilutions of the substance are placed on the patient's tongue. When the proper dilution is found, the patient's symptoms disappear almost instantaneously. Apparently, in these cases, the homeopathic medicine has the ability to affect the general adaptive mechanism so as to counteract the specific symptoms of the allergen extract.

This system, like all such things, has certain limitations, some advantages and several disadvantages. The most important disadvantage is that only a few substances can be tested at a time. It is a time-consuming process which requires a trained professional to observe the patient under the influence of the allergen and select the proper desensitizing dilution. It does, however, pick up fixed allergies, something that some of the other tests described here do not.

Perhaps its greatest use, and the use for which we employ it, is to differentiate from among a few substances which are suspected as being troublesome. If we can narrow down possible sensitivity-producing substances to a dozen or so, the provocative method can be very useful. This test also allows us to develop a specific desensitizing remedy for any substance to which the patient may be sensitive. There can be circumstances in which a patient simply cannot remove himself from an environment to which he is sensitive. With the sublingual provocative test, we are able to discover a desensitizing agent and thus frequently allow the patient to continue in his present employment. The patient would use this agent whenever he comes into contact with the offending substance. None of the other methods of testing has this option. This is now the first test of choice at our Woodlands Healing Research Center.

Food Elimination Diets

A useful method of allergy determination is the elimination diet. Many well-known doctors, such as Dr. Arthur L. Kaslow, of Santa Barbara, California, who is famous for his treatment of multiple sclerosis and similar degenerative diseases, believe that this test is the most practical method of allergy determination.[29] He and other doctors believe that they eliminated technical error by working directly with the patient's physical response. The elimination-diet method is usually pursued by placing the patient on a fast for forty-eight hours and then gradually introducing certain foods which are known to be of a low-allergenic nature. If there is a reaction as food items are added one by one to the diet, the reactive food is noted and eliminated. In the Kaslow method, which is probably the most advanced, this process is continued until twelve foods that the patient can tolerate without symptomatic difficulties are determined. These twelve foods are then rotated in a fashion somewhat similar to the four-day rotation diet. This pattern is continued until the patient shows improvement. As improvement progresses, other foods are added to the rotation pattern as long as they do not cause an adverse effect on the patient's condition.

Airborne Allergens

Because of the development of newer methods, the older skin patch method of allergy testing has fallen into the background with many doctors but it still has many uses, especially for inhaled antigens, including grasses, the common pollens and some of the reactive chemicals. The old skin testing was of little value for food testing, as the accuracy level is low in comparison with the methods already described, but with the development of more sophisticated methodology, skin testing now is an important component of the allergy work at our Woodlands Healing Research Center for airborne allergens.

---

[29] Kaslow, Arthur L., and Miles, Richard B. *You Can Achieve Freedom from Chronic Disease.* Los Angeles, J. P. Tarcher, Inc., 1979.

The influence of airborne allergens on the CFS patient must also be considered. Reactions to airborne allergens can be due to various inhaled substances, such as bacteria, molds, house dust, feathers or pollen. Most of these cannot be eliminated from the environment except by the most drastic measures, such as moving away from an area that may have a high pollen count or having special, expensive equipment installed in the home to keep dust and mold to a minimum. In some cases such measures may be essential to control the allergy, but in most instances supporting the patient's general adaptive mechanism is sufficient to lessen his sensitivity to the allergy.

One item useful in protecting sensitive patients from inhaled allergens is a mask which has proven helpful against inhalants, including common household chemicals and tobacco smoke.[30] The difficulty is to convince patients to use it.

Control of individual particulate matter, *i.e.,* bacteria, small dust particles or pollen, can be maintained by the proper conditioning of the lining mucosa of the nose. This lining contains thousands of little hair-like projections called cilia which are designed to expel any small particulate matter that is harmful to the organism. When working properly, the cilia have an interesting action—they sweep in one direction only. They erect themselves and sweep outward in one motion. On the return motion, instead of sweeping back like a windshield wiper, they become limp and move back slowly, close to the surface of the mucous membrane. In this manner, small particles which might be inhaled and caught by the nasal mucosa are gradually moved to the front of the nares and out by the unique functioning of the cilia.

In many persons who have inhalation allergies, the cilia no longer function properly, and in some cases may be almost functionless. This is yet another effect caused by a breakdown of the general adaptive mechanism and is most commonly seen in patients with rhinitis, sinusitis, postnasal drip and allergies. Upon examining the nasal membranes of these patients, the doctor finds a shiny, glaring red surface rather

---

[30] Manufactured by the E.L. Foust Co., 190 Sunnyside, Elmhurst, IL 60126.

than the pink, velvet-like membrane of the normal mucosa. He realizes at once that the surface has become denuded of cilia, and any foreign particulate substance that enters this individual's nares is easily absorbed into the system since there is no cilia movement to prevent it. This foreign substance is then free to set off an allergic reaction, thus causing no end of trouble and further breakdown in the general adaptive mechanism. As the nares' cilia become progressively less effective, more allergic substances enter the system which further depress the adaptive mechanism which, due to its general weakness, cannot support the mucosa of the nose, and so a vicious cycle is initiated.

Fortunately, an effective treatment now exists for overcoming this difficulty. With this treatment the cilia of most nasal-allergy patients are returned to normal. The treatment consists of two parts: First, patients are put on a low-mucus-forming diet with a special supplement program designed to supply the body with the elements necessary to rebuild the injured mucosa. The supplements contain natural antihistamines and other substances to help control symptoms while the rebuilding process is under way. The second part of the treatment is a unique method of therapy developed by two young eye-ear-nose-and-throat physicians who, in a truly brilliant move, found a way to use a common household appliance to treat one of science's most baffling conditions.[31] In an experiment to find a method of reactivating the nasal cilia, they discovered that if a normal saline solution is pulsed at a specific frequency over the membranes of the nose, the solution stimulates the cilia to action, cleanses the mucus, and helps regenerate the nasal membranes. While searching for an instrument that could be used to pulse the solution, they came upon the standard tooth-cleaning Water Pik.[32] They designed

---

[31] Pope, T., Jr., and Hughes, L. A. Pulsating irrigation: A simple, safe, effective treatment of many nasal complaints. *O. R. L. Digest* 36:10-12, August 1974.

[32] Manufactured by Teledyne Water Pik, 1730 East Prospect Street, Fort Collins, CO 80573.

a special tip for this appliance and tested it on a group of patients. The results were almost universally successful. After perfecting the special tip, which is plugged into the handle of the instrument, they released their discovery to the medical world. While most orthodox physicians find the procedure alien to their normal training and are not inclined to attempt its use, those who have used this appliance have found that it is the most successful instrument yet devised to decongest the nasal membranes and regenerate the cilia. I have seen patients with nasal allergy of many years' standing who have had little relief from other therapies return to a near-normal status within a short time on this therapy. One of the nice things about this treatment is that the patient can use it at home, and thus it is both effective and inexpensive—an uncommon pair today.

Chemical Toxicities

Chronic Fatigue Syndrome can be adversely affected by many types of toxic substances. These can be divided into two main groups: poisonous substances which are completely alien to the system and have a direct destructive effect on the protoplasmic material of the body, and substances that are beneficial in small amounts, but which become toxic to bodily functioning in higher concentrations. The first group can be further divided into those that occur naturally and those that are man-made.

All drugs used in the earlier days of medicine were derived from Nature. Man's skill and expertise had not yet evolved sufficiently to allow him to construct such substances from basic elements. Some of these natural drug substances, such as belladonna and digitalis, and the heavy metals, which will be discussed shortly, are still used today in medicine and can be toxic if not carefully controlled. Fortunately, the CFS patient is usually free of most of the conditions that require use of these naturally occurring toxic substances; however, the possibility of drug toxicity should never be overlooked if a patient seems strangely resistant to therapy.

Several common drugs that are detrimental to CFS patients are used daily by much of the population. CFS patients must stop or severely curtail their use of these drugs if they are to improve. Caffeine has a short-term stimulative effect, but a long-term exhausting effect on the adrenals, and must be eliminated before any real progress can be made. Not only should coffee, tea and cocoa be eliminated from the diet, but also such products as Anacin, No-Doze and all other caffeine-containing over-the-counter drugs. Nicotine, another naturally occurring substance, is decidedly toxic to the CFS patient. Therefore, the smoking and/or chewing—which is not a forgotten art in this country—of tobacco is a "no-no" for CFS patients. These detrimental drugs will be discussed in greater detail later in this chapter.

Foods of the nightshade family (eggplant, peppers, potatoes, tomatoes) have been pointed to as affecting certain arthritic patients adversely. Possibly, because of the alkaloid nature of their components, they may also have a detrimental effect on some cases of CFS. In my experience, this is not necessarily a strong factor, but it should be considered if the more common stresses in an unresponsive patient have been exhausted.

While the above-mentioned naturally occurring toxic elements are important in the treatment of CFS, the body at least has a fighting chance to detoxify these substances to a greater or lesser degree, since these compounds are a part of our ecological environment—we were both created by the same God and came from the same evolution. Man-made organic chemicals, however, are another matter entirely. With these, chemical companies have "for better living through chemistry" created a group of environmental poisons that are unique to our sphere, alien to the basic ecology of the body, and therefore in many instances devastatingly toxic. No doubt they constitute an important factor in the general deterioration of our nation's health. There is not a great deal I need to say on this subject, for authors with far greater skill than mine have written many books on the problems of these man-made toxic chemicals. Some of these substances, such as DDT and TCP and dioxin, have become so infamous that even our sluggishly moving government bureaucracy finally stepped in to limit or discontinue their use entirely.

The profusion of these man-made toxic substances is so great, their distribution so wide and their effects on the human organism so ubiquitous and insidious that only rarely are we able to point to a specific patient and say, "Ah, yes, this is the TCP toxicity." or "This is the BHA toxicity." Man-made organic chemical contaminants are not easily detected because their chemistry is changed once they enter the human body. Their effect on the body is also difficult to ascertain because of the complex nature of the body's enzymatic mechanisms and their interplay with these chemical compounds. It is this indistinct relationship between the absorption of these chemical horrors and symptoms of their toxicity that allows this "greatest of all crimes against humanity" to continue. Because their effects are insidious and subtle and because it is difficult to point to any one substance or manufacturer and say that that substance is the culprit, manufacturers of these death-dealing compounds are able to continue their production until the damage created by their substances has become so obvious that all can see and be affected. By this time, great injury has been done. Even then, when one compound is removed, the manufacturers will produce others to take its place that may have even greater harmful effects, but these will only be discovered at a still later time. So on ad infinitum.

There are only two ways to combat these undiscoverable toxicities. The first is to avoid contact with the toxic substances, and the second is to foster an aggressive program to support those mechanisms in the human body that are designed to detoxify, wherever possible, these destructive compounds. As long as the man-made chemicals are not within man's ecosphere, the adaptive system of his body can, if strong and expertly fortified, provide him with some protection.

At our Centers, we make an exhaustive examination of our patients' dietary intake and general environmental life patterns, suggesting changes we feel will help remove such organic toxins from their foods and general habitat. If the toxic situation is severe, we bring the patient into our Sanctuary and place him in a specially prepared environment that is as free of such toxic contamination as we can make it. At the same time, a special program designed to stimulate and regenerate the detoxifying mechanism of his body is begun. Using these methods, we are able to produce results that have astonished and pleased not only the patients and their families, but also their previous physicians.

Of the enormous amount of disease now present in this country due to the toxic effects of these man-made substances, only a minute portion is treated as such. Most of these effects are being treated as some form of emotional or psychological disorder for which more such organic chemicals are prescribed in the form of tranquilizing agents and antidepressants. Hardly a day goes by in our Center that we do not see pitiful patients who have lost control of their nervous system and have constant involuntary muscular contractions due to long-term use of these tranquilizing agents and antidepressants. Of all the insidious dangers to which we as a people are subjected, this one creates within me the greatest fear. No one knows what long-term effects this multiplicity of man-made toxic substances will produce on future generations. Only within the last sixty or seventy years have we been able to produce such a plethora of alien toxic substances. It will take several generations to even begin to understand the effects such a poisoned world can have on our people. When the final results are in, those well-meaning scientists who perpetrated this travesty will be long in their graves, but wherever they are, if there is justice in the universe, and I'm certain there is, we can but offer for them this prayer, "Lord, forgive them, for surely they knew not what they were doing." The damaging effects on humanity of such men as Genghis Khan, Hitler and Stalin combined must be looked upon as infinitesimal beside the deadly human destruction of such misguided would-be benefactors.

By this time you are undoubtedly asking yourselves, "What can I do to prevent such chemical invasion of my own body?" First, read all labels carefully. Accept nothing with any form of additive unless you know the additive to be safe. Practically no man-made additive is safe, no matter what the Food and Drug Administration may say. Absolutely no one knows enough about the chemistry of the body to know what will happen when we ingest a molecular structure that does not occur in Nature. All man-made substances which are ingested, applied or inhaled by the body must be suspect. All forms of aerosols, hair sprays, toothpastes, antiperspirants, preservatives and colorings must be suspect. There is no such thing as an artificial coloring that is not toxic to some degree. One must go out of one's way to purchase food and drink that is as close to its natural state as possible, as little processed as possible and with as few additives as possible. Any other attitude is self-destructive.

We should work in our communities to reduce environmental poisoning. If each community will control the companies and factories in its own area, then and only then will we have a clean world. There is no industrial production or process that cannot be carried out safely if the people involved are willing to spend the necessary time, energy and inventive skill to do so. However, it will not come about unless we, as an outraged public, demand it. One cannot count on the good intentions of business.

No one is more dedicated to the free enterprise system than am I. I am wholly dedicated to the American dream and the principles of self-determination and personal responsibility. However, when any company, in the name of free enterprise and in search of profits, starts polluting the water I drink or the air I breathe, it has overstepped the bounds of its rights and is infringing upon my rights. I then have not only the right, but a duty to myself, to the company and to my country as a whole to see that it ceases this destruction of our environment. It is incumbent upon us all to do what we can to reduce this chemical exposure to an absolute minimum in our lives and in the lives of those we love. It is also important that we become a voice, a conscience, if you will, for our town, our state, our country to work for laws and programs that will help to reduce and eliminate this chemical contamination. The American dream of opportunity also must carry with it the assumption of certain responsibilities. Unless this is done, it is not a dream—it is a nightmare.

Heavy Metal Toxicity

Among the toxicities that can affect the CFS patient, the toxicity produced by an excess of the heavy metals in the system should never be forgotten. Such heavy metals include copper, lead, mercury, cadmium, nickel, aluminum and arsenic.

Many of the classical philosophers (particularly Paracelsus) had a concept in which they referred to the "microcosm" and the "macrocosm," the macrocosm being the world and universe at large, and the microcosm, man. According to this philosophy, the microcosm is identical to the macrocosm except it is in miniature form. In their view, man has within him every element and substance that is present in the larger macrocosm; the proportions are also similar in that elements rare on earth are rare in the human body. I am not personally adverse to this concept and feel that even in the case of such heavy metals as mercury, lead and cadmium, a minute amount may be useful to the human body. When these small amounts are exceeded, however, serious toxic effects are produced in the system. There is no doubt about this relationship in the case of copper, selenium and nickel. These elements are vital to the functioning of the human body. Recent research in Mexico and in the United States, for instance, has shown that a common type of heart disease present in this part of the world is directly related to selenium deficiency.[33] It is also known that elevated selenium causes specific toxic effects. In

---

[33] Passwater, Richard. *Supernutrition for Healthy Hearts.* New York, The Dial Press, 1977, pp. 112-118.

working with these metallic elements, a tightrope has to be walked to create the proper chemical balances within the body. We need enough, but not too much. If deficiencies occur, certain diseases can ensue; but if excesses occur, toxic effects will be produced that are particularly detrimental to the adrenal patient.

The heavy metal toxins, though not as insidious as the man-made organic chemicals, are an important part of our toxic environment. Fortunately for us, it is possible by the use of tissue analysis to discover these toxicities. Toxic metal poisoning of an acute, massive nature has been known for some time and has been treated by orthodox medical technology. The chronic type of heavy metal toxicity has largely been ignored. However, with the greater perfection of tissue analysis methods available, even the most hidebound, orthodox medical practitioner can no longer afford to discount such toxic problems—which have become an important part of medicine and are an answer to many present medical enigmas. The patient with unexplained symptoms and difficulties who has not been checked for metal toxicity has not had the best of modern medical diagnosis. He should have such tests at his earliest convenience.

Lead

Lead is one of the most common toxic metallic substances with which we deal. Acute lead poisoning may occur in children who eat leaded paint, painters who are daily exposed to this substance, or persons who work in battery factories and other areas where large amounts of lead are utilized. Such massive toxicity is usually detected before the patient comes to us, so we see few of these patients. The best treatment for this condition is EDTA (ethylene diaminetetracetic acid) chelation.

Many chronic lead toxicity cases are found via hair analysis, and as these cases can mimic the symptoms of CFS, they are of great importance. When an elevated amount of lead is found in the hair, we carefully investigate all possible sources of contamination. Where necessary, we make a test of the elements of the patient's environment, such as well water, home-grown fruits and vegetables and other ingested or inhaled substances which may be unique to this person. Certain brands of bonemeal have proven high in lead. It has been my experience that one must look with great diligence for such sources, as often the toxicity comes from the last source one might suspect.

I shall never forget a patient from an ecologically concerned family who had moved to a mountainous area of Pennsylvania to "get away" from industry and contamination and to raise their own fruits and vegetables. After the family had been in the mountains a while, their health gradually started to deteriorate. Heavy metal analysis of their bodily tissues showed an overabundance of lead. Try as we would, we could not discover the source. Finally, in desperation, we asked the state agriculture department to check the levels of heavy metals in their home-grown fruits and vegetables. The amount of lead in this produce was found to be well above accepted levels. After giving up home-grown fruits and vegetables and following a concentrated detoxification program, the family regained health. To this day we are not absolutely sure of the source of the excessive lead in the home-grown produce, but apparently their garden was situated in such a location that as automotive or industrial fumes were blown across their mountaintop, the lead precipitated onto their growing greenery. This example shows the insidiousness of heavy metal pollution of our environment.

The program we use to detoxify chronic lead is as follows: The ingestion of cooked beans (one-half cup daily), vitamin E (up to 800 I.U. daily), B-complex, vitamin C (1000 mg three times daily), vitamin A (25,000-50,000 IU. daily), and the following oral nutritional detoxifying agents: (1) sulfhydryl amino acid-based products (one to three per day, *i.e.,* methionine, cysteine), (2) deodorized, allicin-free garlic preparations (three to six daily), and (3) broad-spectrum fiber products (bran) (three times daily). (See Appendix III for further information about lead toxicity.)

Calcium, zinc, chromium, manganese and selenium also provide protection from chronic lead toxicity. Calcium from nonmilk sources is preferable, however, as milk products can increase lead absorption. The use of distilled water should be considered as long as the essential minerals are replaced during detoxification with a multimineral preparation.

If the condition does not respond to oral medication, as checked by follow-up hair tests, intravenous (EDTA) chelation should be used. In severe cases of lead toxicity, the change in personality after chelation is often dramatic.

Mercury

Mercury, though not as common a contaminant as lead, frequently appears elevated in mineral testing. Such toxicity generally results from the overingestion of tuna or swordfish, but occasionally its cause is cosmetics manufactured with ammoniated mercury. If a patient with high mercury content is placed on a no-tuna diet and the general detoxification regime as suggested above for lead, his mercury level usually drops to normal in a relatively short time. If he, like myself, is a great fish eater, he should eat the smaller fish, for the smaller the fish, the lower the amount of mercury. In my experience, while no heavy-metal poisoning is without its adverse effects, elevated mercury levels do not seem to produce as severe an effect as do elevations of lead, cadmium, aluminum and copper.

In recent years a great deal has been made of the mercury in tooth amalgam fillings and CFS. Some doctors always recommend that the amalgams be removed, while others think it is a useless expense. We tend to take a middle course and have them replaced by less toxic substances only if we find high mercury levels in our patient. The problem we often encounter is that in the removal of the amalgam fillings more mercury is released into the system than was being released previously. Some patients have problems only after the fillings have been disturbed. Therefore, it is a judgment call on the part of the physician whether or not to have mercury fillings removed. At present, many dentists are developing special methods of removing the amalgams that are safe. Most certainly, if you feel you should have your mercury fillings removed, you would do well to seek out one of these specialists. Other sources of mercury toxicity are listed in Appendix III.

Cadmium

Used as a protective covering for metal objects by various industries and in automobile tires as well as in paint, cadmium is a toxic element which has become of greater importance of late. Cigarettes are also a source of cadmium. Most authorities find it difficult to eliminate cadmium as long as a patient is a cigarette smoker. Toxology tests reveal that cadmium, microgram for microgram, is far more toxic than lead. Therefore, in elevated cadmium, every effort should be made to find and eliminate, if possible, the source. These sources, along with some of the toxic effects of cadmium, are given in Appendix III.

Aluminum

Aluminum is another common toxic mineral. The main sources, in our experience, are the aluminum chlorhydrate of antiperspirants, the aluminum trisilicate in various antacids, the aluminum salts in double-acting baking powders which are also present in most over-the-counter bakery goods, and aluminum cookware. The worst offenders are the antiperspirants. For patients with elevated aluminum levels who use these preparations, we recommend they change to one that does not contain aluminum chlorhydrate. These are available through most health food stores. Read the labels carefully, however; recently a recommended brand has added a new aluminum compound to its formula. Aluminum is aluminum. Beware and reject any product with it, no matter the nature of the compound.

Aluminum is toxic to the brain, and the most frequent symptoms of such toxicity are premature senility and loss of memory. These cases are common in our practice; unfortunately, once memory loss and premature senility have set in, it is difficult to reverse the symptoms. However, stringent elimination of all aluminum sources and a careful detoxification program can do much good in these cases. Nevertheless, it is far better to prevent this toxicity than to cure it. The treatment of aluminum toxicity is somewhat more difficult than that of some of the other heavy metals. Several researchers have found beneficial effects with the general detoxification regime recommended under the section for lead plus the addition of homeopathic aluminum in low potencies. (See Appendix III.)

Arsenic and Nickel

Arsenic and nickel are rarely found in elevated amounts in patients. If they are, a careful search must be made for the source, the most usual of which is some form of industrial contamination. Nickel, at times, is found to be high in heavy cigarette smokers. It seems to come from the paper. The cure is obvious. (See also Appendix III.)

Copper

In discussing these toxic metals, I have purposely left copper for last, because its relationship to CFS is substantially different from that of the other heavy metals. Elevations of the metallic substances previously mentioned cause added stress to the system which must be corrected before a complete resolution of CFS is to be expected. They are, however, not by their nature directly connected to CFS. True, elevation of lead and cadmium can cause symptoms which mimic CFS, but this is basically a problem of differential diagnosis, not one in which there is a direct relationship between the disease and the metal levels. This is not true concerning copper. An elevated copper level often indicates a metabolic defect which is directly related to CFS.

The most common hair test pattern observed among CFS patients is one which presents elevated calcium, copper and magnesium levels and depressed sodium and potassium levels. The elevated copper is not essential to this diagnostic pattern, but when it is present, it reveals that the patient has CFS symptoms and that the elevated copper will complicate treatment. Many researchers feel that the mechanism which creates the weakness in the general adaptive mechanism may also create a fault in the body's ability to eliminate copper, and therefore it accumulates in the system. This excess copper can create a symptom pattern which parallels that of the hypoadrenal, creating not only tiredness and exhaustion, but also various forms of bizarre mental and emotional reactions. Dr. Carl C. Pfeiffer and his group at the Brain Bio Center,[34] Princeton, New Jersey, found that patients with this condition often exhibited symptoms similar to those of schizophrenic patients. Our experience confirms these findings.

There are two types of copper toxicity: that which comes from increased ingestion and that which comes from defective elimination. The first type is not necessarily connected with the CFS, but the second is. Patients with either type suffer from high copper levels, but the second much more than the first. In both cases the first essential to treatment is the reduction of copper intake. As far as detoxification treatment is concerned, zinc and manganese, which are antagonistic to copper, are given in large amounts along with a high potency form of rutin, which tends to counteract the adverse effects of copper on the body. These are usually combined with the ingestion of two quarts of distilled water a day for a month to help leech the toxic metal from the system. Such treatment is usually extremely effective, although in certain cases it may have to be continued for several months before it has its required result. (See Appendix III for further information.)

Hair Contamination

Our mineral tests measure elements present in the hair of our patients. It's always possible that the substances we find in the hair may be contaminants and not truly representative of

---

[34] Pfeiffer, Carl C., and the Publications Committee of the Brain Bio Center. *Mental and Elemental Nutrients.* New Canaan, CT, Keats Publishing, Inc., 1975.

the environment within the body. Especially is this true of the toxic metals. It is the policy of our Healing Research Centers to confirm elevated toxic metals found in our hair tests by rechecking with pubic hair. Pubic hair, always (or almost always) being covered, is usually safe from environmental contamination. About half of our toxic head hair readings prove to be contaminated, as evidenced by comparison with normal pubic hair readings. About the only time pubic hair tests fail is in the prepubertal child and in those who swim in pools. To retard algae growth, most pools use copper sulfate that will show in both pubic and head hair. In both of these instances we take retests with finger- and/or toenails.

Miscellaneous Stresses

There is no end to the catalog of stresses that may affect the CFS patient. The list is as long and extensive as the imagination of man himself. Additional stresses which are not well-known, but which have proven to be important causative factors for many Chronic Fatigue Syndrome patients, must be mentioned.

Fluorescent Lights

In the light spectrum of most fluorescent lights certain light frequencies are accentuated, while other frequencies are attenuated. This produces in a graph of these light frequencies various so-called "spikes," sudden spurts of light energy produced within a narrow frequency range. Experiments, reported in such prestigious magazines as *Scientific American,* demonstrated that abnormal light patterns emitted by fluorescent lights are detrimental to the glandular system of the human being, in particular the pituitary gland. These investigators[35-37] discovered that many serious health problems may

---

[35] Painter, Marylyn. Fluorescent lights and hyperactivity in children. An experiment. *Education Digest* 42:36-37, April 1977.

[36] Ponte, L. How artificial light affects your health. *Reader's Digest* 118:131-134. February 1981.

[37] Wurtman, Richard J. Effects of light on the human body. *Scientific American* 233:68-77, July 1975.

ensue from living or working in an environment of fluorescent lighting. The ideal light for man's glandular system, as determined by their research, is daylight. Incandescent light, that is, the regular light bulb, while not equal to daylight, does not have the spikes of the normal fluorescent lighting, and therefore is not as dangerous as fluorescent lights and can be recommended in place of them for indoor lighting.

One of the companies that produces fluorescent lights, DuroTest Corporation, conscious of this problem, has produced a tube known as "Vitalite,"[38] in which every attempt is made to produce a spectrum of light as closely resembling daylight as possible. That they have succeeded may be shown by the fact that their Vitalite can be used as the exclusive light source by which to grow healthy plants. Other companies are now also producing safe fluorescent bulbs and if you desire to obtain some give us a call at 1-800-300-5168.

A patient who is susceptible to CFS may be severely affected by an environment in which he is exposed for long periods to ordinary fluorescent lighting. The best solution for the person who cannot change his employment is to substitute some of the new full-spectrum fluorescent tubes for the ordinary ones. Almost all our patients who have done this have reported improvement in their general health and, in particular, freedom from headaches which had often afflicted them.

Alcohol

Alcohol is basically a vasodilator, which tends to open or dilate the blood vessels. In persons afflicted with CFS, the vascular system is already too dilated by the nature of the disease, and alcohol in any form further aggravates the condition. The Chronic Fatigue Syndrome patient, therefore, should abstain from alcohol totally. Not only does it have a direct adverse effect on his neurohormonal condition, but the lack of control precipitated by its effect on the brain centers often leads the patient to activities that produce compounding

---

[38] Manufactured by the Duro-Test Corporation, 2321 Kennedy Boulevard, North Bergen, NJ 07047.

stresses he would have avoided were it not for the effects of alcohol.

Drugs

Most patients with CFS have been given various drugs by physicians to help allay symptoms which are part of the syndrome. In the long run, the amount of stress induced in the system by the drug usually far outweighs any symptomatic relief received. The most common drugs given are the antidepressants and tranquilizers, either separately or combined. In my experience, until the patient is weaned from these drugs, a total cure of Chronic Fatigue Syndrome is not possible. However, because of the semiaddictive nature of these compounds, care must be taken in the withdrawal procedure. I have seen cases in which we were unable to discontinue tranquilizers for six months because we had to change the patient's unstable, dependent personality before we dared remove his last crutch.

We find, in our practice, that patients often use any form of stimulus they can to realize some relief from the grinding exhaustion and cerebral dysfunction inherent in Chronic Fatigue Syndrome. They guzzle large amounts of coffee, smoke frequently, swallow tranquilizers and mood-elevating drugs in an attempt to give them some semblance of normalcy. Although the effect of these substances is to give temporary succor, they produce a long-term deterioration of the patient's condition, and full recovery is impossible until they are eliminated. Usually they must be withdrawn one at a time. If a patient is on three crutches and we remove all three at once, he will fall flat on his face. It has proven most effective to conquer one habit fully before attempting to work on the second, and so forth.

Coffee

Coffee drinking, like so many habits which afflict mankind, has created much controversy about its constructive or destructive nature among health authorities. Some consider it a mildly stimulating healthful drink. Others have indicted it as a probable cause of heart attacks and strokes. While there is no consensus of opinion as to the general value of coffee drinking, there is a consensus of opinion as to its effect on the CFS patient. Because of coffee's short-term stimulating effect, but long-term debilitating and exhausting effect on the adrenal glands, it is one of the first habits the CFS patient needs to give up if he is to improve. Not only is the caffeine detrimental, but coffee has a specific affinity for the adrenal glands—since even decaffeinated coffee is injurious to the adrenal patient—and must be considered the chemical stress par excellence for these patients. In a patient who uses coffee, alcohol, cigarettes and antidepressant and tranquilizer drugs—a surprisingly common combination in the Chronic Fatigue Syndrome patient—coffee is still the first substance that I suggest be discontinued. Of all of the above-mentioned substances, it has the most direct and profound effect on the adrenal mechanism.

For those who feel that they must have some form of hot drink to take its place, we recommend the cereal "coffees." The ideal substitute, however, is a brew made from licorice root powder obtainable from most health food stores. Properly flavored, this drink is not only tasty, but contains specific substances that have an extremely beneficial effect on the adrenal glands. When the patient substitutes the licorice root tea for his coffee, he manages not only to give up a harmful habit, but also to take on a beneficial one by the same act.

Cigarettes

While few other physicians have mentioned cigarettes per se in regard to CFS, experience has shown us that this common habit also adversely affects the syndrome. CFS patients who smoke improve only up to a point, and no further, until they are able to give up the tobacco habit. Once they abstain, normal improvement again continues until the condition is finally resolved.

The pharmacology of cigarette smoking is not as clear or as well documented as that of coffee. However, it seems to have a somewhat similar effect as this latter substance in that it produces first a short-term stimulation and then long-term deleterious effects to the adrenal gland integrity. The discontinuance of coffee can produce strong withdrawal symptoms in CFS patients, but the avoidance of smoking rarely produces these same effects in CFS. For this reason, as mentioned previously, we usually withdraw coffee first, to remove the greatest stress first before we concentrate on the cigarette habit. In the non-CFS patient the opposite is usually true, but so much is to be fairly easily gained in the Chronic Fatigue Syndrome patient by the elimination of coffee that we give it top priority.

Complicating Conditions

Because of the frequency with which a physician encounters CFS, he must exercise restraint to keep from using this diagnosis too freely. There are other conditions that mimic the adrenal symptoms. Many of these conditions may be found in conjunction with CFS and often require specific treatment before the patient can make the proper progress with CFS. Among these are hypothyroidism, myocardial weakness and B-6 metabolism deficiency.

Hypothyroidism

Lowered thyroid function is frequently induced by the weakened adrenal. This tendency is discovered by the screening blood test made at the beginning of the CFS patient's care. If the physician is still in doubt, the Barnes temperature tests may be made.[39]

If these tests demonstrate a thyroid deficiency, a low dose of Armour dessicated thyroid gland,[40] should be tried. If the diagnosis is correct, the patient should notice improvement in

---

[39] Barnes, Broda O., and Galton, Lawrence. *Hypothyroidism. The Unsuspected Illness.* New York, Thomas Y. Crowell Co., 1976.

[40] Prepared by Armour Pharmaceutical, Executive Office, 303 South Broadway, Tarrytown, NY 10591.

a week or two.

A much superior product made from the fresh thyroid gland, called Proloid,[41] used to be available, but like so many such things the eccentricities of the market or the pressure of the FDA have left it only as a pleasant memory.

Myocardial Weakness

Another condition which can be an added stress to CFS, or a condition by itself, is mild myocardial weakness. The weakness of the heart muscle, or myocardium, may be such that it is not sufficient to cause the classic symptoms of congestive heart disease such as shortness of breath, edema of the extremities and severe exhaustion, but still may cause a lessening of the body's efficiency, mild states of exhaustion and other symptoms which closely mimic those of CFS. While the more severe of these patients can be detected by careful analysis of their electrocardiographs, the EKGs of many of the milder cases of myocardial weakness do not deviate far from normal; therefore, the milder cases may not surface during a usual examination. In our Center, careful analysis of the heart using a sensitive phonocardiograph (an instrument that records the sounds of the heartbeat on a graph, rather than the electrical potentials as does the EKG) discloses most of these cases, since the weakening muscular contractions of the heart are displayed quite accurately.

Patients with this condition have benefited from using glucoside-rich nontoxic herbs to support the heart action. The best combination is a remedy which contains one part *cactus grandiflores* to five parts *crataegus oxacanthus*. This remedy not only is useful and harmless, even when given over a long period of time, but also has proven to be an excellent tool for the differential diagnosis of this condition. Whenever I have a borderline case, not certain if the heart is involved, I test the patient by giving the proper dose of the *cactus–crataegus* mix-

---

[41] Prepared by Parke-Davis Division, Warner-Lambert, 201 Tabor Road, Morris Plains, NJ 07950.

ture for one month and then discontinue its use for the same period. If the patient improves in strength and general functioning ability during the "on remedy" period, but begins to regress a week or two after the discontinuance of the herbal remedy, it is a positive sign that he has a minor degree of myocardial weakness. Since the *cactus–crataegus* mixture is completely nontoxic and well accepted by the sensitive systems of most CFS patients, it should be used as a therapeutic test if there is any question that a CFS patient might have a weakened myocardium (heart muscle).

B-6 Metabolic Defect

Two recent tests have been added to our repertoire to allow us to measure a new factor in human nutrition: the mauve factor test and the X-K procedure. Both of these tests measure an excess of waste produced because of B-6 deficiency, dependency or malassimilation. These products are porphyrins in the mauve factor test and xanthurenic acid and kynurenic acid in the X and K test.[42-43] The mauve factor (or kryptopyrrole) often is found in the urine of patients with adrenal dysfunction as well as in patients with mental disorders. Deficiency of vitamin B-6 causes excessive spillage in the urine of the X and K acids which indicates a blockage in the pathway of the conversion of the amino acid tryptophane to the neurotransmitter serotonin.

The products of B-6 metabolism are vital to proper brain functioning. If they are deficient, the mind is fuzzy, depressed, and in many ways similar to that encountered in CFS. Since we do not as yet know the exact defect in metabolism that causes this unavailability of the B-6 metabolites, we must treat this condition by supplying the end products of this breakdown, pyridoxal-5 phosphate and L-cystine. When these are supplied, the metabolic defect is circumvented, and the brain

---

[42] McCabe, Donald Lee. Kryptopyrrole in clinic practice. *Osteopathic Medicine* September 1980, pp. 43-59.

[43] Sauberlich, H. E., and others. *Laboratory Tests for the Assessment of Nutritional Status.* Boca Raton, FL, CRC Press, Inc., 1979.

once again receives the food it so desperately requires. If this malabsorption has been of long duration, it can take some time before the brain can recover its integrity, but perseverance with the remedies will be rewarded. It is not known whether CFS is the cause of this effect, but the frequency with which it is found in these cases is certainly suspicious.

Summary

Many environmental factors create stress in the CFS patient—factors of which the patient may not be aware. Included are infective states, allergies, chemical toxicities and miscellaneous stresses. Among specific infections which may have untoward effects on the CFS patient are acute and chronic infections, of which *Progenitor cryptocides* and *Candida albicans* can be especially deleterious. Allergic reactions may now be tested in a number of ways, and methods have been devised for protecting against airborne allergens. Heavy metal toxicities may affect CFS patients—including toxicity to lead, mercury, cadmium, aluminum, arsenic, nickel and copper. Miscellaneous stresses may be caused by fluorescent lighting, alcohol, coffee, drugs, cigarettes or by complicating conditions such as hypothyroidism, myocardial weakness or B-6 metabolic defects.

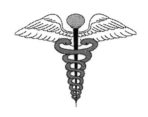

Chapter Eleven

Sex and the CFS Patient

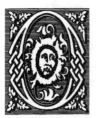NE of the questions I am often asked by CFS patients and their families is, "What about sex for those with this condition?" Over the years, my findings have shown that a dispirited sexual life is one of the most frequently encountered stress-creating problems among persons afflicted with CFS. Although a cursory description of what I mean by a dispirited sex life is included here, an in-depth explanation of this subject is given in our recent work, *One Flesh*.[1] For those interested in further information on this fascinating subject, we highly recommend *One Flesh* from this publisher.

As detailed in *One Flesh*, three factors must be present for sexual activity to create a sustained beneficial and constructive effect on the human organism:

> 1. There must be a physical exchange of both the male and the female sexual fluids at each coitus. This exchange must be made without chemical substances in the vagina which might be detrimental to the activity or absorption of either the male or the female discharges.[2]

---

[1] Poesnecker, G.E. *One Flesh*. Quakertown, PA, Humanitarian Publishing Co., 1996.

[2] This was originally written before the AIDS plague was upon us. However, the statement is still valid if we are to expect the benefits Nature and our Creator meant us to derive from the sexual (Continued on next page)

2. There must be strong feelings of love, not lust, or mere sexual attraction, between the copulating couple, or there can be produced in the sexual fluids of one or the other toxic components that are harmful to the physical and emotional health of both parties. This is particularly true for the woman who is inclined to CFS.

3. There must be a willingness on the part of both participants to accept full responsibilities for the consequences of their act. They must not only accept the possibility of pregnancy in those individuals who are of the appropriate age bracket, but they must also accept the responsibility for one another. Through the combining of sexual life fluids, they have become one person. The Biblical phrase is "and they twain shall become one flesh." If these responsibilities are not accepted, then an insidious, almost unconscious form of guilt develops which, in my experience and that of many other dedicated investigators, eats at the core of human neurohormonal integrity, sometimes causing, but always aggravating CFS.

(Continued from the previous page) union. The popular wisdom today is that to have "Safe Sex," one must always have some latex or plastic wrap between the two parties, and at no time are they to exchange bodily fluids of any kind. While this may or may not prevent the spread of AIDS it certainly will prevent any of the positive, constructive effects that are a normal part of the sexual union from taking place. If I really enjoyed treating CFS patients, I would be jubilant over this doctrine since I have little doubt that it will help produce a vast new number of patients with CFS. However, if the truth were known, I would be deliriously happy if all CFS patients were normal once again so that I could really retire and enjoy my golden years as others do. But my sense of duty is such that I will keep up my crusade until I am satisfied that CFS patients are being given the care and attention they need to truly regenerate.

To these three factors may be added a fourth that, though not a primary requirement for neurohormonal sexual stability, is an added bonus to those who are desirous of deriving the greatest possible benefit from their sexual forces. By special training, it is possible for a couple to use their sexual powers to improve and heal diseases and weaknesses of the body. Admittedly, this procedure is little understood and even less practiced in the modern world, but it is available to all who desire it and can be a most marvelous adjunct in the regeneration of those who have a weak general adaptive mechanism.[3]

To those members of the Christian faith who have been taught that the sexual function per se was the "original sin," it must seem heresy to consider sex as a beneficial or constructive act. However, the mere fact that many consider sex the "original sin" and wish it would just go away does not change in the slightest the true nature of sex or its great potential to affect the human organism for good or evil. Sexual congress per se was *not* the original sin. The original sin, and in truth, as taught by the ancient philosophers, the beginning of all sin, was the *misuse and abuse* of the sexual function. Many knowledgable physicians still hold that such misuse and abuse of the sexual function remains the greatest single cause of disease, misery and emotional instability in the world today.[4]

That the abuse of the sexual function has the power to degrade and degenerate is little disputed by most of mankind. The very words "degenerate" and "debauchery" carry with them strong sexual connotations. A very lucrative component of organized crime is devoted to supplying degenerate sexual activity to our people, be it in the form of male or female prostitution, pornography, or any other form of licentious sexual activity which might be turned into an unholy dollar.

---

[3] This method is described in detail in *One Flesh.*

[4] As mentioned, this was written before the AIDS epidemic. Today these words seem almost prophetic. The honest doctor asks the question, "What will be the consequences of the 'sterilization' of sexual activity by the 'Safe Sex' procedures?" If we accept the thrust of this chapter, are we not to question whether the "Safe Sex" cure is not more deadly than the disease?

We all are familiar with this dark side of sex, but is there another, equally potent compensating side of light and health?

From our observation of Nature, we notice that none of its inherent forces are either good or evil. Only the direction and application of these forces make them constructive or destructive. The greater and more universal the force, the greater power it will have wherever it is directed. If it is directed in an evil way, the destruction shall be great. If, on the other hand, it is directed in a constructive manner, the effect can be as beneficial as the destructive would be harmful.

Sex, as any other force in Nature, is just that—a force, a power, a potentiality. It is only the manner of its use that determines whether its effects will be good or injurious. If we acknowledge that the sexual function has great potential for the degeneration and destruction of man's physical, emotional and moral fiber, we must agree that the converse is also true; that properly used and directed, sex has an equally strong potential to uplift and regenerate man's physical, emotional and moral being. Any other conclusion would be counter to the reality of our natural world.

We have all been given many gifts by our Creator, but none is greater than our sexual potential. The use we make of it determines its effect for good or ill upon us and upon those who become a part of our responsibility. If we accept this simple fact of life, it behooves us to learn the laws of our own sexual functioning, to attempt to live according to these laws, and constantly to strive to further develop their use for constructive and regenerative purposes. As we do this, we will have conquered one of the greatest problem areas of human life, and our days will be long and joyous.

The Three Laws of Constructive Sex

First Law: Exchange

It is an absolutely essential requirement for any sexual, regenerative process that there be an adequate, uncontaminated exchange of male and female secretions during the sexual embrace. It is amazing how often this God-ordained requirement is neglected and/or misunderstood by society as a whole and by physicians in particular. As described in *One Flesh,* the male and female fluids contain many complex organic substances in addition to the basic reproductive cells. These hormonal and nutrient factors are vital to the integrity of the neurohormonal mechanism of both male and female. They are particularly important to the female, as the male nervous system is as a whole less fine and less highly organized than that of the female.[5]

Any form of sexual activity or method of birth control that prevents this proper exchange of fluids on a reasonably regular basis will prove detrimental to any married woman, whether or not she has CFS. If women who have this condition are sexually aroused, but are not given the necessary male fluids to absorb vaginally, their neurohormonal systems can experience a devastating shock.

A few moments' reflection will recall to mind that several common forms of birth control and/or sexual activity prevent this necessary physical exchange and can create this neurohormonal havoc. Any form of sexual activity that produces an ejaculation outside the vagina prevents this essential exchange. The use of any type of protective sheath, *i.e.,* condom, surrounding the male organ during intercourse also precludes any such exchange. Various forms of chemical suppositories, spermicides and even the ineffectual, but commonly used douche following intercourse are detrimental by either physically removing the health-giving substances or by neutralizing portions of them through chemical action.

For those for whom contraception is important, there still remain several effective methods that do not interfere with this exchange. On a purely mechanical level, two of the more

---

[5] There is a saying, "It doesn't matter if the crock hits the rock or the rock hits the crock; it's the crock that always suffers." So it is with sex and the woman; with her more finely tuned nervous system, she is the one who pays the most in a sexual union without normal fluid exchange.

modern methods of birth control—the birth control pill and the intrauterine device (IUD)—do not interfere with this sexual exchange. Unfortunately, both of these methods have other detrimental effects which may lead the intelligent, conscientious woman to seek elsewhere for a method of contraception. The pill inclines toward various hormonal imbalances and increases the chance of serious vascular difficulties.[6-8] The IUD has a nasty habit of burrowing into the vaginal wall, causing various forms of infection and often necessitating complicated surgical removal.[9-10] Recent research has also shown that infection with *Actinomyces* bacteria is now common in women who leave an IUD in over long periods.[11-13] This infection can cause a disagreeable pelvic infection which frequently leads to infertility.

---

[6]Pfeiffer, Carl C., and the Publications Committee of the Brain Bio Center. *Mental and Elemental Nutrients.* New Canaan, CT, Keats Publishing, Inc., 1975. Chapter 48.

[7] Ambrus, J. L., and others. Progestational agents and blood coagulation. VIL Thromboembolic and other complications of oral contraceptive therapy relationship to pretreatment levels of blood coagulation factors. Summary report of a 10-year study. *American Journal of Obstetrics and Gynecology* 125:1057-1062, August 15, 1976.

[8] Beral, V., and others. The pill and circulatory disease. *American Heart Journal* 97:263-264, February 1979.

[9] Zakin, D., and others. Complete and partial uterine perforation and embedding following insertion of uterine devices. II. Diagnostic methods, prevention and management. *Obstetrics and Gynecology Survey* 36:401-412, August 1981.

[10] Connell, E. B. Side effects of IUDs. *International Journal of Gynaecology* 15⁽2⁾:153-156, 1977.

[11] Burkman, R., and others. Relationship of genital tract actinomycetes and the development of pelvic inflammatory disease. *American Journal of Obstetrics and Gynecology* 143:585-589, July 1, 1982.

[12] Drew, N. C. Genital and pelvic actinomycosis. Case report. *British Journal of Obstetrics and Gynaecology* 88⁽7⁾:776-777, July 1981.

[13] Gupta, P. K., and others. Actinomycetes and the IUD: An update. *Acta Cytology* (Baltimore) 22:281-282, September October 1978.

Two other methods that allow successful sexual exchange, but that do not have the adverse systemic effect of the contraceptive pill and the IUD, are the diaphragm and the so-called rhythm method. Admittedly, neither of these is perfect, there being no such thing at this time, but when properly used, they can be effective in birth control without deterioration of the sexual exchange.

For those whose religion or personal conviction does not forbid it, we generally recommend the use of a properly fitted and utilized diaphragm. By "properly utilized," I refer to the fact that in our Centers, we suggest that contraceptive jelly be used only on the inside of the diaphragm (that part which goes directly against the cervix) and that a nonspermicidal jelly, such as K-Y,[14] be used for the rim of the diaphragm. In this way, essential fluids do not come in contact with any spermicide and are thereby not chemically altered. Purists will undoubtedly contend that a certain portion of the vaginal wall is covered by the diaphragm and can therefore not excrete the feminine fluid nor absorb the masculine fluid, as is required. Admittedly, this is true. Approximately one-third of the vaginal wall is covered in this manner. However, long experience by physicians knowledgeable in the process of sexual regeneration has shown that sufficient secretion and absorption do occur in the remaining two-thirds of the vagina to allow full benefit to be gained from the sexual exchange. The physical and emotional benefits gained by preventing pregnancies that the couple may not be adequately able to support more than offsets any minor fluid deprivation that might come from the use of the diaphragm.

As a couple grows older and their secretions and absorbing ability begin to diminish, the ability to create new life also diminishes, and finally contraception is no longer necessary. At this time, when increased absorbing area is desirable, the entire vagina becomes available for secretion and absorption.

Those whose religious conviction does not allow use of the diaphragm must depend on methods which restrict inter-

---

[14] Prepared by Johnson & Johnson, New Brunswick, NJ 08903.

course to times when the egg is not present for fertilization. Many age-old counting techniques have been suggested and they work for some but not others. In more recent times, advanced methods such as the use of basal temperatures are available to help find these periods of infertility more accurately than in the past. Such methods are at best difficult and undependable; however, there is certainly no impediment to the proper sexual exchange, and where religion decrees or the couple desires no mechanical device, there is no other alternative. Some women are more regular than others, and therefore much more likely to have success with this method of birth control. If this is religiously or morally the only method open to you, I highly recommend that you consult a physician who is well trained in this procedure and follow his advice as closely as possible.

One last subject to be discussed is abstinence. Many newer religious groups advise their adherents that the only practical method of birth control is abstinence. While admittedly this method is effective, it is usually detrimental to the neurohormonal systems of both the male and the female. The laws laid down by our Creator for the use of the sexual function are right use, not abuse or nonuse. For all individuals, but particularly for those with lowered neurohormonal functioning, the exchange of sexual fluids carried out under the proper circumstances is one of the greatest life-regenerating factors known to mankind. The end result is the same whether this exchange does not occur because of perverted sexual habits or because of abstinence from sexual activity. If there is no exchange of sexual forces, there is no exchange—whether from the use of "Safe Sex" or abstinence. You cannot make something from nothing. Abstinence is not an answer for those who are married. The benefits of sexual regeneration are available only to those who use the sexual function constructively and productively.

Many may wonder about individuals who never marry or who are divorced or widowed. Are these ofttimes well-meaning people kept from the beneficial forces of sexual regeneration? The answer is both yes and no. Yes, in that since they have not accepted the responsibilities of marriage, they have no rights to the benefits of the state. Sexual regeneration is one of the major benefits of accepting the responsibility of a home and family. Any attempt in this matter, as in all of man's endeavors, to obtain the benefits without assuming the responsibilities would be breaking the Laws of Nature and of God.

The answer to this question is also "no," however, as these persons are not denied the benefits of sexual regeneration. There is another manner in which those who are single can use the sexual forces for their own constructive and regenerative purposes. This method, described in our book *One Flesh*, is of such complexity that it is not practical to repeat here. However, for those interested, I again recommend this earlier text, or better yet, suggest that those sincerely interested make an appointment at our Healing Research Center for a personal consultation on this matter.

Second Law of Sex: Love

While the first tenet of regenerative sex use is somewhat revolutionary, at least it is easier to explain and understand than the second and third laws. The second law, which insists on love between the two parties who participate in the sexual union, at first may seem to be based on some ancient and unexplained religious dictum or on some romantic fantasy. Actually, neither is the case. The requirement that love be present is based on pragmatic functioning of the human body and is completely explainable in physical terms.

While the first tenet concentrates on quantitative factors, the second is concerned with qualitative factors. In other words, the first tenet is concerned with the mere physical exchange of the male and female sexual secretions. We assume that these substances will be beneficial. Unfortunately, this assumption cannot always be made. It is a foregone conclusion among advanced endocrinologists that various secretions of the human body can be altered by the mental and

231

emotional status of the individual, and compounds which under normal circumstances would be beneficial and sustaining can become injurious and toxic if produced in an environment of disturbed human emotion.[15-16]

While this is a very complicated matter, it is sufficient for our purposes to state that if one of the parties to the act of love holds within himself or herself resentment, envy, hatred or any other adverse emotional feeling toward the sexual partner, the secretions which that person contributes to the sexual exchange can be detrimental to both parties concerned. While we have not heretofore considered the fact, there is always the possibility that a child may be conceived from such a congress, and when such emotional disharmony exists, one must wonder what kind of stability will be built into the fiber of this child. "A bad tree cannot bear good fruit."

Married CFS patients often have a variety of problems which may alter the qualitative nature of the sexual fluids involved in exchange. Most frequently, the nature of CFS itself tends to lessen sexual desire, especially in women. This lack of desire can produce a tendency toward abstinence when it occurs in the man, but when it exists in the woman, it can have various adverse effects on the marriage act. If the woman's husband is kind and understanding, he will not force himself upon her, and therefore the result is greatly lessened frequency, which tends to produce a physiological withering of the sexual function, and of course little or no sexual regeneration. In these patients a tremendous force for rebuilding health and overcoming CFS is therefore neglected.

If the husband is not so thoughtful and tends to force his personal desires on his wife, several consequences may occur. Having no great personal desire for the sexual act, she may merely "let him have his way with her," assuming that this is part of her duty as a wife. However, she does not enter into the

---

[15] Clark, Blake. Your emotions can make you ill. *Reader's Digest* 100: 129-132, May 1972.

[16] Jonas, Gerald. Manfred Clynes and the science of sentics. *Saturday Review* 55:42-46, May 13, 1972.

spirit or pleasure of the act, not so much because she wouldn't like to, but because she is just too tired to create the necessary initiative. Such negative acceptance produces a low quality of sexual fluid exchange.

Other wives in this situation may feel that their husbands take advantage of their masculine position and force upon them something in which they really have no interest. Therefore, they build within their hearts a resentment toward their husband's actions and toward sexual activity as a whole. This resentment prevents them from producing constructive sexual fluids and prevents a proper absorption of the husband's fluids, and so while the physical exchange may take place, the quality or the spirit of the exchange is so poor that it can create a detrimental rather than a constructive effect on both parties. Often in these instances, especially when the CFS patient is a young woman, her husband is rapidly turned off by her attitude and either looks elsewhere for a sexual outlet, or the couple retreats into a state of voluntary abstinence. Either scenario prevents the wife from obtaining the needed benefits of sexual regeneration to help her overcome her problem.

Ideally, the sex life of those with CFS must be lovingly cultivated. Neither abstinence nor force is the answer. The couple must understand and consider the eccentricities of the CFS patient, but also practice, when and where possible, sexual regeneration. As this is done, the CFS will improve and more frequent sexual regeneration can be instigated. In this, as in most things, "Love conquers ALL."

Third Law: Responsibility

Of all the tenets, the third is the most difficult to delineate and substantiate. This does not reduce its importance, and it is just as important as the others in constructive and creative sexual regeneration.

Man is not merely an animal. He is half god, half animal. This unique combination within one being produces a creature who is physically capable of doing all the heinous acts his mind can imagine, but also creates in him a conscience that can drive him to extremes of despair and depression over the actions of his uncontrolled animal nature within. Most of us have within us a strong sense of natural justice. Although our human desires may drive us to commit acts counter to the Laws of God and Nature, we know deep down that we are doing wrong and will condemn ourselves through the conscience. The guilt that is produced causes a stress that is difficult for the most skilled of counselors and physicians to exculpate.

We realize that there are those human beings who are seemingly without conscience or guilt. Many of these merely hide it from their fellowman, but within them there is a gnawing and burning which allows no true rest. Admittedly, there are those who truly are without conscience, and who are unaffected by right and wrong, what is just and what is unjust, or what is fair and what is unfair. These people cannot be reached. They are outside the mainstream of civilization. They are pure animal and are devoid of the spark of God possessed by the normal human. We can only protect ourselves and those we love from these nonhumans. The great majority of people do have a conscience, however, and do feel guilt when they break the Laws of God and Nature.

To understand this tenet of sexual responsibility, one must first understand our Creator's plan for sexual health. The basic plan for man's sexual activity is simple, and all evaluation of such activity must be made in direct comparison with the scenario determined by our Creator. Allegorically, when God created Adam, He looked at him and said, "It is not good for man to be alone," and He forthwith created woman. This was one of God's first acts—that of creating the sexual components of humanity—man and woman. Later He laid down the dictum that these two should join and that the twain, that is the two, should become *One Flesh*. The whole act of marriage, but particularly that part of it relative to the sexual exchange, has the capability of making this man and this woman one being, or as the Bible says, "One Flesh." They become a single human functioning unit. This is the essence of God's plan, the apogee of one part of the creative function.

Ideally, soon after the awakening of the sexual desires in both the male and the female, the Creator planned that the young man and woman should find one another and join together on a lifelong journey in which they would raise a family, establish a home as a training ground for this family, and become a strong, powerful functioning unit that would work for the good, not only of themselves and their family, but of all humanity. They would exercise the sexual desires the Creator gave them without any interference in the sexual exchange or without any attempt to use the sexual organs in any manner that does not allow for proper exchange as described in the first law. They would engage in the sexual embrace only when they felt strong love for one another and would never engage in it when there was anger, jealousy, hatred or resentment within their hearts. By the nature of their love and honesty, they would assume full responsibility for one another, caring for one another "in sickness and in health, for better or for worse, for richer or for poorer," because they had in truth become one person. As such, "that which God has joined together, let no man put asunder."

This is the God-given ideal of human love, marriage and sex. The closer a human couple is able to come to this ideal, the better will be the chance of using their sexual functioning for regenerative or healing purposes. The further they deviate from this ideal, the less chance they have of succeeding at sexual regeneration.

Admittedly, in this day and age not too many couples fit into this category of an ideal relationship. However, this in no wise changes the fact that such an ideal relationship can exist, and still is God-ordained as ideal for His human creatures' lives. The fact that such an ideal is so rare does not show that God is at fault, but only how far we have deviated from the way He would have us go. In any marriage, the amount of guilt created is inversely proportional to the amount of responsibility which the partners of this relationship are willing to assume. Many people today are living with or having sexual relations with individuals who wish to enjoy the sexual and other advantages of such a relationship, but are not willing to take upon themselves the responsibilities of a true marriage and family. This weakness of character produces subliminal guilt feelings that are a cancer within the system and can destroy the contentment and emotional stability of either or both parties.

All modern protestations to the contrary, in only one way can a man demonstrate his true commitment to the responsibilities inherent in the beneficial use of the sex act, and that is by legally accepting the responsibilities of marriage. Any other modern sophistry is only so much seductive hogwash.

It is an unfortunate human trait that most of us are always looking to obtain something for a price less than its real worth. The price of sexual activity and regeneration is the acceptance of each and every responsibility that may accrue from such an involvement. This includes the responsibilities toward the other person involved, toward the children that may come from such a relationship, plus all the other moral and legal responsibilities inherent in producing a home and family.

From time immemorial, men particularly have done everything within their power to sidestep this responsibility while still enjoying the pleasures of sex. Only within recent years, however, have they been so seductive in their arguments that they have been able to convince women that the unmarried state also has advantages for the fair sex. This accomplishment must win the prize as the greatest bit of chutzpah ever to take place in the world! It obviously is the greatest job of salesmanship of all time.

I have counseled thousands of individuals who are attempting to live a sexually active life without assuming the God-ordained responsibilities of marriage. I have yet to find one who could even approach the contentment and stability of the sexually regenerate life lived according to the Laws of God and Nature. Mankind, it seems, will do everything within its power to avoid doing that which is right and just, and as a consequence has brought itself to an unprecedented state of weakness and degeneration—physically, mentally and emotionally. CFS is only the tip of the iceberg here, and we have little doubt that it will be followed by many related conditions of weakness in the years ahead.

Regenerative Sex

I have often been accused of being a harbinger of doom by telling people what was wrong with the sexual activities of modern life and not telling them how to overcome these difficulties. I hope in part to overcome this reputation by discussing as much as I may how the sexual function may be utilized to help bodily regeneration generally and the CFS patient in particular.

When the individual desirous of sexual regeneration is married, every effort should be made to engage in the sex act at least once a week. Twice a week is to be preferred if circumstances and the health of both parties allow. Relations more frequent than this are not detrimental unless they are forced and unappreciated by one of the couple.

If contraception is necessary, a diaphragm should be fitted and used according to the method described previously, unless religious tenets preclude its use—in which case, the patient should confer with a physician well versed in the rhythm method of birth control.

Every effort should be made to develop the love between those participating in the sex act.[17] This act should not be consummated if there is resentment, jealousy, envy, loathing, hatred or any other adverse emotion between either of the partners. If such feelings do exist, they should be talked out before the sex act takes place. If they can be resolved and the feelings of love between the two once again established, the sex

---

[17] One of my editors (a woman) asked in her note to me, "Have you ever heard of 'foreplay'? I haven't seen you address this in your books." My books are not meant to be "sexual manuals" but rather to be a spiritual extension of such texts. However, I will say that I agree with the French who state, " The art of love is the art of pleasing the woman." To the wise man this means not only a good knowledge of foreplay but also practical skill in its application.

act may proceed. However, if the adverse feelings between the couple cannot be resolved, the act should be postponed until such a state of love can once again be achieved.

Whenever possible, an individual should not get trapped into so-called "relationships" in which all the benefits of marriage are expected with as few of the responsibilities assumed as possible. Such "relationships" are little more than the modern equivalent of the kept mistress with all of the disadvantages of that situation and very few of its advantages.

The purpose of this instruction is to keep sex from becoming a stress, to prevent it from having a negative effect on the CFS patient. There is, however, a more important and fascinating aspect of the sex function. That is its use as a healing therapy. It can become a treatment method as potent as any we have in overcoming many chronic ailments, including CFS.

To be used for healing purposes, one must first fulfill the three primary tenets of sexual activity. When these are followed, a person can, during the rest periods of the sexual act and during the period following the conclusion of this act, command his body to direct these infused energies to the healing purpose desired. In the case of CFS, during the rest periods of the sex act and during that period following the sexual climax, both partners should hold in their minds and hearts this thought, "We are desirous of utilizing as much as possible these energies which we are exchanging during this act of love, to help build and strengthen my body (her body/ his body), to help overcome the weakness in my (her/his) neurohormonal system." The words obviously do not have to be the same as these, but the thought and spirit should be.

Admittedly, many will scoff at the ability of such a naive procedure to be helpful, but if they only knew the inherent powers in the creative centers of men and women and the power of the human mind to direct the forces within its domain, they would realize that such use of the sexual forces is in full accord with Natural and Divine Law, and that such healing has a power which is not exceeded by any other known to man.

Summary

Although sexual activity may be a major stress for some Chronic Fatigue Syndrome patients, when the sexual function is used constructively, that stress can be greatly mitigated. Sex can be a constructive force if three basic laws are followed during the sexual union: First, there must be an adequate, uncontaminated exchange of male and female secretions. Second, there must be love between the two persons who participate in the union. Third, there must be responsibility for the consequences of the union. When these three laws are obeyed, a more important aspect of the sexual function may be brought into being—as a healing therapy—which can become a force for good not exceeded by any other known to man.

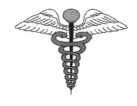

Chapter Twelve

A Few Final Words

HERE can be little doubt today that Chronic Fatigue Syndrome, also known as Adrenal Syndrome, is a viable, demonstrable condition. Nor is there doubt in my mind, after observing and cataloging its effects for nearly half a century, that the number of its victims is increasing exponentially with each passing day. Harold E. Buttram, M.D., in his book *Vaccinations and Immune Malfunction*,[1] expressed the opinion that one of the major causes of this proliferation may be infant malnutrition (not the lack of food, the lack of the proper nutrient rich food) and the assault to the immune system by the multiple vaccinations given early in life. If his conclusions are correct, and the evidence in his book is difficult to refute, it is hard to explain how any of us are able to escape this energy-sapping condition.

For instance, if a child who may have inherited a tendency toward weak adrenals from his parents is brought up on the now-popular commercial infant formulas—which are severely deficient in natural food value—the adrenal weakness has little chance to improve. If his already crippled immune system is then assaulted by the injection of multiple vaccines into his bloodstream (bypassing his natural defenses), his immune system is forced to expend much of its essential

---

[1] Buttram, Harold E., and Hoffman, John Chriss. *Vaccinations and Immune Malfunction.* Quakertown, PA, Humanitarian Publishing Co., 1982

reserve vitality to build antibodies for diseases that sanitation and modern health habits eliminated long ago.

As a young child he is ready prey to every virus that comes his way, and he is usually afflicted with a variety of ear and other upper respiratory infections. For these he is given antibiotic after antibiotic, effectively preventing his body from building normal immune antibodies with what is left of his immune potential. By the time this child enters school and is exposed to the multitude of viruses encountered there, he is frequently a ready victim, due to the fact that many of his defense units have already been committed by the previous vaccines and are not available.[2]

Should such a child be so lucky as to survive to puberty, the added stresses on his glandular system at this time are usually the final blow to the adrenal. In a real sense he never really becomes a whole normal person, but is crippled by adrenal gland weakness before he reaches adulthood. A prime candidate for Chronic Fatigue Syndrome.

Unfortunately, this history is not theoretical. It is the exact story I have heard from thousands of patients. Once this scenario has been enacted it *can* be reversed, but only by great

---

[2] As shown in Dr. Buttram's book, *Vaccinations and Immune Malfunction*, according to the one cell–one antigen rule, once an immune body (plasma cell or lymphocyte) becomes committed to a given antigen (vaccine element), it becomes incapable of responding to other antigens or challengers. In the use of the multiple vaccines usually given in childhood, great sections of the immune cells are forced to be committed to the injected antigens (vaccines). These cells can then never again be used by the body to fight any other disease than those now committed. This would not be bad except it has been shown that the vaccination method is extremely wasteful of the immune cells and many more cells are required to produce immunity by vaccination than are required by natural immunity. It must also be remembered that many of the diseases for which children are vaccinated are not ones usually encountered today. But our antiquated vaccination system, more political than medical, forces the immune system to waste many valuable cells, thereby leaving the child with a lowered defense against the real enemies he will meet along the highways of life.

efforts on the parts of the doctor and the patient as described in this work.

"Why," you ask, "do not more individuals have CFS if it is caused by the circumstances you describe? Certainly, most of us in middle life have had experiences similar to the one you mention."

The reason more individuals do not have CFS is that their immune system and adrenal glands are strong enough to absorb the abuse and still allow them to function in a fairly normal fashion. The problem is that as we go through the generations, the newer generations become weaker than the previous ones and eventually, unless radical changes are made in our medical care, weak adrenals and immune systems will be the norm rather than the exception.

Chronic Fatigue Syndrome is no myth. It is one of the more common consequences of our modern unnatural life. Too long have we, as a society, assumed that we could abuse the fiats of Nature and God without feeling the result of our disobedience.

Our bodies contain marvelous systems for repair and protection, but unless we wake up and learn to respect and husband them, we will soon find that it is not, as now, a minority who have CFS, but the majority. Should we allow this to happen, we as a nation would fall easy prey to those peoples of the Earth who, like the Huns of old, have followed the more natural laws of life.

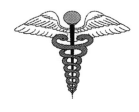

Appendixes

Appendix I: Diets for CFS Patients

Diet #1—Basic Health Maintenance Diet
(For those *without* concurrent hypoglycemia)

This diet, if followed faithfully, will aid in restoring health where lost, and in continuing good health in those so blessed.

First thing upon arising take a full glass of warm water with a pinch of sea salt added. Half a lemon may also be added if troubled with constipation. One half hour later breakfast is taken. Salt may be omitted for persons on a low-sodium diet.

Breakfast #1

Only fruit is taken. One may use as much as desired. The following are particularly recommended: Apples (juice, raw, baked, or as sauce), apricots, bananas (very ripe), berries of all kinds (best raw), cantalopes, cherries, grapefruit (Indian River brand best)*, grapes, lemons*, limes, oranges*, papayas, peaches, pears, pineapples, coconut (fresh best, drink milk), plums, rhubarb*, tangerines*, melons of all kinds. Dates, prunes, figs and raisins may be used if they cause no trouble, but they are more sugar than fruit and should be restricted during colds, flu, and so on. All fruit should be well washed and preferably rinsed in one of the products, sold at health food stores, to remove chemical sprays. If at all possible, try to

---

*These foods should not be used if you have arthritis, bursitis or related diseases.

buy fruit from a private party or health-food source so that it is without sprays. One of the following may be added to this breakfast, if desired or felt necessary: Nuts, seeds, lean fish or meat. These supply sustenance to the meal without disturbing the digestion.

Breakfast #2 (Nonfruit)

Although a fruit breakfast is recommended, some may find it insufficient at first, or they may wish some diversification. The following may be used in this case:

> Cereal: Any whole grain product may be used: Wheatena, steel-cut oats, millet, seven-grain cereal, and other such products.

> Milk or Cream: Raw milk or cream is preferred. Some may be used on the cereal and the rest drunk. Cereal coffee or herb teas may also be used.

> Bread: Whole wheat toast, whole wheat or corn meal muffins, whole wheat waffles, pancakes or cornbread may be used. (Undegerminated cornmeal.)

> Raw Vegetables: Raw vegetables may be and should be taken with the foods above because they are all acid-forming and raw vegetables are needed to control this condition. Raw celery or carrots are sufficient.

Dinner and Supper

Dinner and supper both have similar construction. One meal, either dinner or supper, as the case may be, will be smaller than the other, but the types of foods used are not altered, only the amounts.

Protein

Have only one protein at each meal. (Small portions of two proteins from the same group may be used.) Proper proteins may be chosen from the following:

Group I Dairy Products: Milk (raw), buttermilk, home made ice cream. Cottage and natural cheese (no processed cheese), eggs (fertile if possible) soft boiled, scrambed, or raw. (If you have problems with congestion, use only the yolk.)

Group II Meat or Fish: Lean beef, lamb, chicken, turkey, duck, and all organ meats. (If possible, obtain meats from private parties who do not use chemicals in the animal feed or sodium nitrate as a preservative. Some health food stores also carry naturally produced meat.) All forms of fish are good; those from the sea are richer in essential elements than the fresh water fish, however. All types of seafood (clams, shrimp, crab, etc.) are highly recommended as long as their purity of source and processing is assured. Fish and seafood contain less toxic substances than the meats.

Group III Nuts and Legumes: Nuts, lentils, dried peas, beans, and seeds (sunflower, sesame, etc.) may be utilized but with caution, as they are difficult to digest. They must constitute the only starch or protein taken at the meal.

Starches

Have only one starch at each meal. More than one leads to overeating. Health-building starches should be chosen from the following:

Whole wheat bread made only from the most natural ingredients. Either make your own or use a whole grain bread from one of the health food stores. A nutritious bread is one of the most important articles of diet; be sure yours is the best.

Aside from the staple bread, the following carbohydrates are recommended: baked potatoes, natural brown rice, unpearled barley, millet, steel-cut oats and any products made from natural unrefined grains, *i.e.*, corn bread, whole wheat pancakes, waffles, bran muffins.

Fats

A small amount of fat is useful in most diets. Choose from: Real butter, soybean-lecithin spreads such as are found in the better health food stores. In cooking only the following products should be used: cold pressed oils, such as peanut, soy, safflower, sunflower and sesame. For solid shortening, butter or the above soybean spread may be used. These fats may be more expensive than those in usage today, but they may prevent diseases that could cost a thousand times more.

Vegetables

The rest of the meal should consist of vegetables. It is best if they comprise at least one-half the bulk of the meal. This instruction will help to normalize body chemistry. The following comments apply to vegetables: One half of the vegetables should be raw; if you can eat something raw, do not cook it. If at all possible, try to obtain vegetables that have not been sprayed with pesticides or grown with chemical fertilizers. Your best vegetables are those fresh from the garden— yours or a friend's. Canned and/ or frozen are allowed, but are second best. Each meal should start with a raw vegetable; this is vital. Tomatoes and/ or cucumbers should not be eaten with regular meals, only with other vegetables, meat or fish, not with starches or dairy products.

Additional Instructions

Some products used in preparation of food are necessary but harmful. More healthful substitutes are available and should be used. A list of these follows:

Baking powder: Use only Royal, Rumford, or special health food brands containing no aluminum salts.

Table Salt: Use sea salt from health food stores.

Cornstarch: Arrowroot flour or rice polishings.

Chocolate: Carob candy and powder

White sugar, syrups, etc.: Use only turbinado, uncooked honey, sorghum, Grandma's molasses, maple syrup, and maple sugar.

Desserts: Cakes, pies, cookies, etc., can be made from unrefined foods but should be served as the starch for the meal and not afterward, as is usually done.

Coffee, tea: Use the alkaline herb teas, *i.e.,* Alfa-mint, fenugreek, shave grass, clover, rose hips, dandelion coffee, etc.

All foods should be simply prepared. When spices are omitted from the diet, soon the natural flavors of food prevail and our senses can appreciate their delicate but distinctive nature. Natural spices in moderation are not condemned, however.

Do not eat fruit with regular meals, only for breakfast or as a snack between meals and at bedtime.

Nuts, dried legumes, soy beans can be used by those whose digestion allows. They must constitute the only starch or protein taken at a meal.

Do not, under any circumstances, drink fluoridated water or use it in food. Buy bottled water if necessary.

Diet #2—For Chronic Fatigue Syndrome Patients With Concurrent Hypoglycemia

NOTE: This diet is only a guide; your doctor may not permit some of the listed items.

Upon Arising:	½ half grapefruit
Breakfast:	1 egg with or without 2 slices of meat or fish (no ham or bacon) Only ½ slice of bread or toast, with plenty of butter. Beverage (herb tea or cereal coffee)
2 Hours after Breakfast:	A snack of shrimp, raw nuts or slices of roast beef
Lunch:	Salad (large serving of lettuce, tomato, vinegar and oil dressing) Vegetables if desired Only ½ slice of bread or toast, with plenty of butter Beverage (herb tea or cereal coffee)
2 Hours before Dinner:	A light snack of raw nuts, cheese or celery stuffed with cheese.
Dinner:	Soup if desired (not thickened with flour) Vegetables Liberal portion of meat, fish or poultry Beverage (herb tea or cereal coffee)
Every 2 Hours until Bedtime:	A small handful of nuts or another desired protein.

NOTE: Baked potatoes or rice may at times be substituted for bread unless the condition is severe.

Avoid Absolutely:

Alcoholic and soft drinks such as club soda, dry ginger ale, whiskey and liquors

Sugar, candy and other sweets such as cakes, pies, pastries, sweet custards, puddings and ice cream

Caffeine—ordinary coffee, strongly brewed tea and beverages containing caffeine

Spaghetti, macaroni, noodles, donuts, jams, jellies, marmalades (starch and sugar)

Wines, cordials, cocktails and beers (alcohol is high in carbohydrates)

Hydrogenated fats, partially hydrogenated fats, and fried foods

Allowable Oils: Butter, virgin olive oil, sesame oil, linseed oil (food grade, not boiled)

Four-Day Rotation Diet[1]

Day One

Food Families:

Citrus:	Lemon, orange, grapefruit, lime, tangerine, kumquat, citron
Banana:	Banana, plantain, arrowroot (musa)
Palm:	Coconut, date, date sugar
Parsley:	Carrots, parsnips, celery, celery seed, celeriac, anise, dill, fennel, cumin, parsley, coriander, caraway
Beet:	Beets, spinach, swiss chard, lamb's quarters (greens)
Pepper:	Black and white pepper, peppercorn
Herbs:	Nutmeg, mace
Cashew:	Cashew, pistachio, mango
Bird:	All fowl and game birds including chicken, turkey, duck, goose, guinea, pigeon, quail, pheasant,eggs
Tea:	Comfrey tea (Borage family), fennel tea
Oil:	Coconut oil, fats from any bird listed above, butter
Sweetener:	Use sparingly: Date sugar, orange honey (if honey is not used on another day of rotation), beet sugar
Juices:	Juices may be made and used without adding sweeteners from the following: Fruits: Any listed above in any combination Vegetables: Any listed above in any combination desired, including fresh comfrey
Grains:	Wheat
Fish:	Salmon, tuna

---

[1] Patients may wish to make their own rotation diets. The four-day diet presented here is given to show how it can be done. The basic requirement is that menus be prepared for four days so that a food on the menu on one day is not included on the menus of the three intervening days.

Day Two

Food Families

Grape:	All varieties of grapes, raisins
Pineapple:	(Juice pack, water pack, or fresh)
Rose:	Strawberry, raspberry, blackberry, dewberry, loganberry, young berry, boysenberry, rose hips
Melon:	(Gourd) Watermelon, cucumber, cantaloupe, pumpkin, squash, other melons; zucchini, acorn squash, pumpkin, or squash seeds
Mallow:	Okra, cottonseed
Pea:	(Legume) Peas, black-eyed peas, dry beans, green beans, carob, soy beans, lentils, licorice, peanut, alfalfa
Subucaya:	Brazil nuts
Flaxseed:	Flaxseed
Mollusks:	Abalone, snail, squid, clam, mussel, oyster, scallop
Crustaceans:	Crab, crayfish, lobster, prawn, shrimp
Tea:	Alfalfa tea, fenugreek
Oil:	Soybean oil, peanut oil, cottonseed oil, butter
Sweeteners:	(Use sparingly) Carob syrup, clover honey if honey is not used on another day
Juices:	Juices may be made and used without added sweeteners from the following:
	Fruits or berries: Any listed above in any combination desired
	Vegetables: Any listed above in any combination desired including fresh alfalfa and some legumes
Fish:	Sardines, kippers, halibut
Grains:	Corn, millet
Red meat:	Beef, veal

Day Three

Food Families:

Apple:	Apple, pear, quince
Mulberry:	Mulberry, figs, breadfruit
Honeysuckle:	Elderberry
Olive:	Black or green or stuffed with pimento
Gooseberry:	Currant, gooseberry
Buckwheat:	Buckwheat
Aster:	Lettuce, chicory, endive, escarole, artichoke, dandelion, sunflower seeds, tarragon
Potato:	Potato, tomato, eggplant, peppers (red and green), chili pepper, paprika, cayenne, ground cherries
Lily (onion):	Onion, garlic, asparagus, chives, leeks
Spurge:	Tapioca
Herb:	Basil, savory, sage, oregano, horehound, catnip, spearmint, peppermint, thyme, marjoram, lemon balm
Walnut:	English walnut, black walnut, pecan, hickory nut, butternut
Pedalium:	Sesame
Beech:	Chestnut
Salt-water fish:	Sea herring, anchovy, cod, sea bass, sea trout, mackerel, swordfish, flounder, sole
Fresh-water fish:	Sturgeon, herring, whitefish, bass, perch
Tea:	Kaffir tea
Oil:	Safflower oil, butter
Honey:	(Use sparingly) Buckwheat, safflower, or sage honey (honey can be used if it has not been used any other day)
Juices:	Juices may be made and used without added sweeteners from the following: Fruits: Any listed above in any combination desired Vegetables and herbs: Any listed above in any combination desired
Red meat:	Lamb, mutton
Grains:	Rice, wild rice

Day Four

Food Families:

Plum:	Plum, cherry, peach, apricot, nectarine, almond, wild cherry
Blueberry:	Blueberry, huckleberry, cranberry, wintergreen
Pawpaw:	Pawpaw, papaya, papain
Mustard:	Mustard, turnip, radish, horseradish, watercress, cabbage, kraut, chinese cabbage, broccoli, cauliflower, brussel sprouts, collards, kale, kohlrabi, rutabaga
Laurel:	Avocado, cinnamon, bay leaf, sassafras, cassia buds or bark
Sweet potato:	Sweet potatoes or yams
Grass:	Oats, barley, rye, cane, sorghum, bamboo sprouts
Orchid:	Vanilla
Protea:	Macadamia nut
Birch:	Filberts, hazelnuts
Conifer:	Pine nut
Fungus:	Mushrooms and yeast (brewer's yeast, etc.)
Bovine:	Milk products—butter, cheese, yogurt, milk products, oleomargarine
Tea:	Sassafras tea or papaya leaf tea, lemon verbena tea
Oil:	Butter
Sweetener:	(Use sparingly) Cane, sugar, sorghum, molasses. Avocado honey if honey is not used on another day
Juices:	Juices may be made and used without added sweeteners, from the following: Fruits: Any listed above in any combination desired Vegetables: Any listed above in any combination desired, including any of the tea herbs, obtained fresh

Candida albicans Diet

(Strict yeast and mold avoidance list)

FOODS PERMITTED	FOODS OMITTED

Beverages:

Home-squeezed juice of peeled fruit, cow and goat milk, spring water, tap water — Alcohol, chocolate drinks, coffee (regular and decaffinated), sodas, tea (black and herbal), canned or frozen juices

Breads, cereals, grains:

NO grain products — All grain products are to be avoided

Dairy products:

Butter, eggs, cow and goat milk and plain yogurt — Cheeses, ice cream, margarine, flavored yogurt, sour cream, tofu, buttermilk

Fish and seafood:

Tuna in water, all other fish and seafood that is not breaded such as bass, bluefish, carp, clam, codfish, crab, flounder, haddock, halibut, herring, lobster, mackerel, oyster, pike, perch, swordfish, salmon, sardine, scallop, shrimp, smelt, trout, whitefish, etc. — Tuna in oil, breaded fish or seafood of any kind

Fruits:

Apple, avocado, banana, grapefruit, lemon-lime, nectarine, orange, peach, pear, pineapple, plum, tangerine. All fruit must be fresh and peeled. All fruit has yeast on its surface and should be peeled. — Blackberry, blueberry, cantaloupe, cherry, date, fig, grape, honeydew melon, prune, raspberry, raisin, strawberry, watermelon

Foods Permitted	Foods Omitted
Meats and poultry:	
Beef, chicken, duck, lamb, beef liver, pork, turkey, veal	Fried or breaded meats, hot dogs, cold cuts, gravy
Nuts:	
None	All
Vegetables:	
Beet, cabbage (peel off outer leaves), carrot, cucumber, eggplant, lettuce (peel off outer leaves), onion, parsnip, potato (sweet and white), pumpkin, radish, squash, tomato, turnip. All vegetables have yeast on the surface and should be peeled.	Artichoke, asparagus, broccoli, brussels sprouts, cauliflower, celery, com, endive, green pepper kidney beans, kohlrabi, leek, lentil, lima beans, mushrooms, black olives, parsley, green peas, pimento, red pepper, rhubarb, soy beans, spinach, string beans
Miscellaneous:	Avoid monosodium glutamate and Accent seasonings, herbs, spices

Additional Information

Some individuals are unusually sensitive to yeasts and molds. For such persons, a trial diet which eliminates all foods and drinks that contain yeasts or molds is suggested.

Persons on this diet should keep a food and symptom diary for at least two or three weeks to help spot any changes and/or unsuspected infractions. In the beginning, the diet must be adhered to 100 percent. Then patients may be able to ease up on the diet and discover how strict they need to be to control symptoms.

All sugars and artificial colors, flavors and preservatives are to be avoided on general grounds as well as to simplify the picture for this yeast/mold elimination diet.

ALWAYS READ LABELS CAREFULLY

Most of the following items contain yeasts or molds:

1. All grains, such as wheat and corn, have small amounts of yeast or mold on their surfaces. Flours and cereals are often enriched with B vitamins that are usually derived from yeast. Also leavening or baker's yeast is often added to grain products: Breads, rolls, biscuits, buns, pretzels, crackers, cookies, cakes and pies.

2. All nuts and seeds, dried fruits, teas (black and herbal), herbs and spices (such as cinnamon and pepper) have yeast or mold on their surfaces.

3. Cheeses of all kinds, including cottage cheese, sour cream, tofu and buttermilk contain mold. Plain yogurt is acceptable.

4. Yeast is present in all fermented beverages: all alcoholic beverages, medications containing alcohol and root beer and ginger ale.

5. Most condiments contain vinegar or other fermentation products: catsup, mayonnaise, salad dressings, barbeque sauce, tomato sauce, soy sauce, miso, tamari sauce, mincemeat, horseradish, sauerkraut, olives and pickles.

6. Malt products contain some yeast: malted milk and some cereals and candies.

7. Mushrooms and truffles are mold foods.

8. Many vitamins contain or are derived from yeast. Check the labels and if in doubt, ask.

9. Antibiotics are often derived from mold cultures. If in doubt, ask.

Appendix II: Toxicities in Our Environment

Aluminum

HE toxicity of aluminum has long been a disputed subject. Although many scientists did not previously consider aluminum to pose a significant health risk, recent evidence seriously questions this conclusion. Research now suggests that aluminum may interfere with normal body functioning at levels lower than previously assumed, and there have been increasing reports of aluminum toxicity from environmental exposure.

Sources

Aluminum cooking vessels, baking powder (aluminum sulfate), aluminum-containing antacids, deodorants and antiperspirants, aluminum dust from industrial aluminum manufacturing, building construction materials, household and industrial utensils, insulated cables and wiring, packaging materials (*e.g.*, aluminum foil), fine aluminum powder used in bronze paint, aluminum cans, drinking water (alum used to kill bacteria), soil (naturally occurring ores), coal burning plants including those used as food, beer, milk, and milk products (from equipment), alum used in food processing-pickles, maraschino cherries, medicinal aluminum compounds used externally to treat dermatitis, wounds, and burns, nasal spray (alum), toothpaste, ceramics (made from A1 203 clay), dental amalgams, cigarette filters, tobacco smoke, automotive exhausts, pesticides, animal feed, FD&C color additives, vanilla powder, table salt and seasonings, bleached flour, American cheese, fumigant residues in foods (aluminum phosphide), Kaopectate® and other medications containing kaolin (aluminum silicate), feldspar and mica, McIntyre aluminum powder (used in prophylaxis of silicosis), aluminum silicate paste (arthritis treatment), sutures with wound-healing coatings containing aluminum, aluminum chelates of polysaccharide-sulfuric acid esters for peptic ulcer treatment, aluminum nicotineate (hypercholesterolemia treatment).

Occupational Exposures

Manufacturing of aluminum abrasives, treating bauxite ore to obtain alumina, production of aluminum sulfate (alum) from bauxite ore, manufacturing of aluminum products, aluminum alloy manufacturing, paper industry, glass industry, textile industry (waterproofing), use of aluminum abrasives in many industrial operations, manufacturing of aluminum metal powders, synthetic leather manufacturing, aluminum welding, porcelain industry, explosives manufacturing, pyrotechnical devices manufacturing and use.

Signs and Symptoms

Aluminum pneumoconiosis (inhalation of Al dust): pneumothorax, pulmonary fibrosis with emphysema, dyspnea, right-sided cardiac hypertrophy, Shaver's disease: cough, substernal pain, weakness, fatigue, bilateral lace-like shadowing on lung x ray; phosphate binding in gastrointestinal tract-aching muscles, rickets, osteoporosis; skin reactions (from Al antiperspirants), miliaria (acute inflammation of sweat glands); encephalopathy, senile dementia (Alzheimer's disease), nephritis, hypatic dysfunction, gastric distress, GI inflammation, flatulence, acid eructation (belching), colitis, hyperactivity in children, psychosis in children.

Arsenic

Arsenic is a common environmental contaminant derived from natural and anthropogenic sources. Both oral ingestion and inhalation of arsenic are modes of intoxication. Arsenical toxicity is highly dependent on the chemical form, oxidation state and route of exposure. Natural concentrations of arsenic in foodstuffs are usually rapidly absorbed, but also quickly excreted. Absorbed arsenic is transported by the blood to the kidneys, liver, spleen, skin, hair and nails in that order. Some arsenic may remain in tissues long after it has disappeared from the blood, urine and feces.

Sources

Rat poisons, insecticide residues on fruits and vegetables, herbicide residues on cottonseed products, wine (if arsenical insecticides used in vineyards), drinking water, well water, seafood, some kelp supplements, seawater, feed additives (poultry and livestock), coal burning, air polluted by arsenic dust from industrial plants, wood preservatives, wallpaper dye and plaster (containing volatile arsenicals), Paris green (arsenic containing pigment formerly used in ornaments, toys, curtains, carpets), some household detergents, colored chalk, automobile exhaust.

Occupational Exposures

Smelter workers, chemical workers handling inorganic arsenic, vintners working with arsenical insecticides, sheep dip workers using sodium arsenite, gold miners (associated arsenic ores), processors of taconite (low-grade iron ore), acetylene workers, alloy makers, aniline color workers, bleaching powder makers, boiler operators, bookbinders, bronze makers, colored-candle makers, canners, ceramic enamel workers, painters, paperhangers, petroleum refinery workers, plumbers, solderers, tree sprayers, wood preservative makers, hide preservers, taxidermists, weed sprayers, forestry workers.

Signs and Symptoms

Headache, drowsiness, confusion, brittle nails, follicular dermatitis, hoarse voice, Raynaud's phenomenon (poor circulation to extremities), weakness and muscular atrophy, palmar and plantar keratoses, pigmented spots on trunk, atypical (precancerous) keratoses on hands, feet, and trunk, squamous cell carcinoma of skin, "Mees lines" (transverse white ridges or parallel lines on nails), erythromelalgia (burning pain, redness, swelling of hands and feet), hemiplegia, sensory changes (parathesias, hyperesthesias, neuralgias, myalgia), garlic odor on breath and perspiration, goiter, heart failure, hypertension, hepatomegaly and jaundice.

Cadmium

Cadmium is toxic to every bodily system whether ingested, injected or inhaled and tends to accumulate in body tissues. Consequently, there is concern about the increase in environmental cadmium that has occurred as a result of its increasing industrial use. Inhaled cadmium is usually better absorbed than ingested cadmium. Once absorbed, the elimination rate is generally very slow. The toxicity of cadmium, however, is significantly influenced by dietary intake of other elements such as zinc, copper and selenium.

Sources

Drinking water, soft water, causing uptake of Cd from galvanized pipes, soft drinks from vending machines with Cd piping, refined wheat flour (increased Cd:Zn ratio), evaporated milk, many processed foods, oysters, kidney, liver, rice (irrigated by Cd-contaminated water), soil, cigarette smoke, tobacco, superphosphate fertilizers, Cadmium alloys (*e.g.,* dental prosthetics), ceramics, paint pigments, electroplating, cadmium-vapor lamps, tools rustproofed with cadmium, marine hardware rustproofed with cadmium, welding metal, solders, silver polish, polyvinyl plastics, fungicides, pesticides, sewage sludge and effluents, copper refineries, dust in urban streets, homes, businesses and schools, rubber carpet backing, wear of rubber tires, burning of motor oil, plastic tapes, black polyethylene, black rubber, nickel-cadmium battery manufacturing, zinc or polymetallic ore smelting, paint manufacture using cadmium pigments, painting with cadmium pigments, jewelry making, cadmium alloy manufacturing, ceramic making using cadmium, electroplating metals with cadmium, process engraving, cadmium vapor lamp manufacturing, rustproofing tools, marine hardware, soldering, tetraethyl lead manufacturing (uses diethyl cadmium), fungicide manufacturing.

Signs and Symptoms

Fatigue, hypertension (possibly related to increased concentration of Cd in renal parenchyma), iron-deficiency anemia, emphysema, Itai-Itai (osteomalacia in parous women over forty years of age with dietary deficiencies), slight liver damage, anosmia (loss of sense of smell), yellow coloring of teeth, reduced birthweight in newborns, renal colic (with passage of calculi), nephrocalcinosis, hypercalcuria, pain in lower back and legs, pain in sternum, "Milkman's syndrome" (lines of pseudofracture in scapula, femur, ileum), hypophosphatemia, possible rheumatoid arthritis, decreased production of active vitamin D, decreased pulmonary function, proteinuria, glucosuria, and aminoaciduria (following nine years of inhaling Cd oxide), possible prostatic cancer (in workers exposed to Cd oxide), possible carcinogenesis, increased mortality.

Copper

Although copper is an essential element, there are situations in which the possibility of human copper toxicity requires consideration. Wilson's disease (an inborn error of human metabolism) represents a special case of copper toxicosis. Large amounts of copper accumulate in the liver, kidney and brain of those with this disease. Copper can be absorbed by the lungs, skin, uterus and gastrointestinal tract. The toxic effects of copper are related to the adequacy of other elements, such as zinc.

Sources

Drinking water, copper plumbing and piping, surface and ground water, animal and industrial waste, fungicides and insecticides, sewage sludge, oysters, liver, nuts, chocolate, vinegar, carbonated beverages or citrus juices if prolonged contact with copper, beer (from copper piping and brew kettles), refrigerator ice makers, hemodialysis, copper intrauterine contraceptive devices (IUDs), copper in dental prostheses, milk (accumulates copper from heated copper rollers during pasteurization), industrial emissions, swimming pools (fungicide), copper cookware, vitamin-mineral supplements.

Signs and Symptoms

Accidental poisoning (acute): vomiting, diarrhea, jaundice, impaired liver function, hemoglobinuria, hematuria, oliguria, hypotension, coma, death; copper metal fume fever: chills, fever, aching muscles, dryness of mouth and throat, headache, digestive disorders; arthritis, scleroderma, eczema, schizophrenia, postpartum psychosis, autism, gingivitis (caused by Cu-containing dental work), nasal irritation, bitter taste, anemia (iron deficiency), atherosclerosis.

Lead

Lead has long been known as a toxic element. At one time it was believed that the only significant sources of increased lead ingestion were plaster, paint or industrial exposure. Although this is probably true for acute lead poisoning, it is not true for chronic lead toxicity. The increasing prevalence of lead as an environmental contaminant has led to subclinical exposures which often result in subtle, yet significant, adverse health effects. Lead may enter the body through ingestion, inhalation or skin eruption. Adults normally absorb 5 to 10 percent of ingested lead, while children may readily absorb up to 50 percent. Inhaled lead is absorbed at 25 to 100 percent, depending on the lead particle size. Tolerance to lead varies with age, form and source of the lead and with the composition of the diet being consumed.

Sources

Atmospheric lead-motor vehicle exhausts, lead smelters, coal burning, refining lead scrap, burning materials containing lead; dust and dirt, leaded house paint, drinking water, lead plumbing, vegetation growing by roadside, vegetables grown in lead-contaminated soils, canned fruit and fruit juice, canned evaporated milk, milk from animals grazing on Pb-contaminated pastures, bonemeal, organ meats, especially liver, lead-arsenate pesticides, wine (leaded caps), rainwater, snow, improperly glazed pottery, painted glassware, pencils (paint), toothpaste, newsprint, colored printed materials, spitballs, eating utensils, curtain weights, putty, car batteries, cigarette ash, tobacco, lead shot, mascara, painted children's toys, PVC containers, canned pet food, hair dyes (progressive darkeners).

Occupational Exposures

Acid finishers, actors, battery makers, blacksmiths, bookbinders, bottle cap makers, brass founders, brass polishers, braziers, brick burners, brick makers, bronzers, brushmakers, cable makers, cable splicers, canners, cartridge makers, chemical equipment makers, chlorinated paraffin makers, chippers, cigar makers, crop dusters, cutlery makers, decorators (pottery), demolition workers, dental technicians, diamond polishers, dye makers, dyers, electronic device makers, electroplaters, electrotypers, embroidery workers, emery wheel makers, enamel burners, enamelers, enamel makers, explosives makers, farmers, file cutters, firemen, flower makers (artificial), foundry workers, galvanizers, garage mechanics, glass makers, glass polishers, gold refiners, gun barrel browners, incandescent lamp makers, ink makers, insecticide makers, insecticide users, Japan makers, Janers, jewellers, junk metal refiners, kiln workers, labelers (paint can), lacquer makers, lead burners, lead counterweight makers, lead flooring makers, lead foil makers, lead mill workers, lead miners, lead pipe makers, lead salt makers, lead shield makers, lead smelters, lead stearate makers, lead workers, linoleum makers, linotypists, linseed oil boilers, lithotransfer workers, match makers, metal burners, metal cutters, metal grinders, metal polishers, metal refiners, metal refinishers, metallizers, mirror silverers, musical instrument makers, nitric acid workers, nitroglycerin makers, painters, paint makers, paint pigment makers, paperhangers, patent leather makers, pearl makers (imitation), pharmaceutical makers, photography workers, pipe fitters, plastic workers, plumbers, printers, policemen, pottery glaze mixers, pottery workers, putty makers, pyroxylin-plastic workers, riveters, roofers, rubber buffers, rubber makers, rubber reclaimers, scrap metal workers, semiconductor workers, service station attendants, sheet metal workers, shellac makers, ship dismantlers, shoe stainers, shot makers, silk weighters, slushers (porcelain enameling), solderers, solder makers, steel engravers, stereotypists, tannery workers, television picture tube makers, temperers, textile makers, tile makers, tinners, type founders, typesetters, vanadium compound makers, varnish makers, vehicle tunnel attendants, wallpaper printers, welders, wood stainers, zinc mill workers, zinc smelter chargers.

Common Nonoccupational Lead Exposures

Ceramics, pottery and related hobbies, stained glass work, electronics and related hobbies involving extensive soldering, firing ranges, hunting (especially those who cast their own bullets), eating or drinking (from improperly fired lead-glazed ceramic tableware), eating lead-bearing paint, burning battery casings, consuming illicitly distilled whiskey, extensive auto driving (especially in cities), extensive work with motor fuels, painting with lead-containing paints, home plumbing repairs (lead pipe systems), exterminating.

Signs and Symptoms

Headache, depression, insomnia and/ or drowsiness, fatigue, nervousness, irritability, dizziness, confusion and disorientation, anxiety, muscle weakness and wasting, saturnine gout, aching muscles and bones, abdominal pain, loss of appetite, loss of weight, constipation, hypertension, kidney function defects, reproductive defects, decreased fertility in men or spontaneous abortion in women, impaired adrenal gland function, iron-deficiency anemia, blue-black lead lines near base of teeth.

Symptoms More Common in Children

Hyperactivity, temper tantrums, withdrawal, frequent crying for no apparent reason, fearfulness, refusal to play, other emotional or behavioral problems, drowsiness, learning disabilities, speech disturbances, perceptual motor dysfunctions, mental retardation, seizures or convulsions, ataxia, encephalopathy.

Mercury

Mercury, long known as a toxic element, has evoked increasing concern in recent years because of its increasing use in industry and agriculture and the burning of fossil fuels. Methylmercury compounds and elemental mercury vapor are the two forms most likely to be involved in human exposures. In addition, the conversion of elemental mercury and mercury compounds by bacteria to the more toxic methylmercury also poses potential threats to human health. Ingested methylmercury is readily absorbed through the gastrointestinal tract and inhaled mercury vapor is easily retained by the pulmonary system. Skin absorption of mercury may also occur.

Sources

Mercury-silver amalgam (dental fillings), broken thermometers and barometers, consumption of grain seeds treated with methylmercury fungicide, fish and marine mammals, mercuric chloride (used in histology laboratories), calomel (body powders and talcs), mercury-containing cosmetics, latex and solvent-thinned paints, organic mercurials (diuretics), air polluted by industrial mercury vapor, mercury-polluted industrial water, clothing worn by mercury workers, hemorrhoid suppositories using mercurials, Mercurochrome and Merthiolate (thimerosal), fabric softeners, floor waxes and polishes, air conditioner filters, wood preservatives, cinnabar (used in jewelry), batteries with mercury cells, fungicides for use on lawns, trees, shrubs and so on, tanning leather, felt, adhesives, laxatives (containing calomel), skin-lightening creams, psoriatic ointments, photoengraving, tattooing, laboratory and industrial equipment using metallic mercury, sewage sludge used as fertilizer contaminates soil, sewage disposal (may release thousands of tons of Hg annually world wide).

Occupational Exposures

Amalgam makers, bactericide makers, barometer makers, mercury battery makers, boilermakers, bronzers, calibration instrument makers, percussion cap loaders, carbon brush makers, caustic soda makers, ceramic workers, chlorine makers, dental amalgam makers, dentists, direct current meter workers, disinfectant makers, disinfectors, drug makers, dye makers, electric apparatus makers, electroplaters, embalmers, explosives makers, farmers, fingerprint detectors, fireworks makers, fish cannery workers, fungicide makers, fur preservers, fur processors, gold extractors, histology technicians, ink makers, insecticide makers, investment casting workers, jewelers, chemical laboratory workers, fluorescent lampmakers, Manometer makers, mercury workers, mercury miners, mirror makers, neon light makers, paintmakers, papermakers, percussion cap makers, pesticide workers, photographers, pressure gauge makers, mercury refiners, seed handlers, silver extractors, mercury switch makers, tannery workers, taxidermists, textile printers, thermometer makers, vinyl chloride manufacturers, wood preservative workers.

Signs and Symptoms

Elemental mercury vapor exposure: insomnia, shyness, nervousness, dizziness, loss of memory, lack of self-control, irritability, anxiety, loss of selfconfidence, drowsiness, depression, loss of weight, loss of appetite, tremors; severe cases: hallucinations, manic depression; organic mercury exposure: earliest symptoms—fatigue, headache, forgetfulness; later findings—numbness and tingling of the lips and feet, muscle weakness progressing to paralysis, loss of vision, hearing difficulty, speech disorders, loss of memory, incoordination, emotional instability, dermatitis, renal damage, general brain dysfunctions; late symptoms—coma, death.

Nickel

Nickel can be a toxic element in man. It can interact by four routes of entry into the body. These are oral ingestion, inhalation, parenteral administration and percutaneous absorption. Nickel or nickel salts are relatively nontoxic when taken orally. Nickel toxicity from parenteral administration has only been observed experimentally. Percutaneous absorption may manifest as nickel dermatitis and is relatively common. The inhalation of nickel carbonyl causes the most serious type of nickel toxicity, although it usually occurs only in occupational workers due to an industrial accident.

Sources

Stainless steel cookware (Ni taken up by acid foods), tobacco smoke, contamination of air, drinking water, soil, and vegetation by industrial nickel, testing of nuclear devices (radionuclide Ni-63), exhausts of automobiles and trucks, burning of coal and oil for power generation, burning of fuel oil for space heating, wear of automobile tires and brake linings, superphosphate fertilizers, dissolved nickel from food-processing equipment, hydrogenated fats and oils, baking powder, nickel-cadmium storage batteries.

Sources of Contact for Allergic Individuals

Nickel jewelry, nickel coins, clothing fasteners, tools, cooking utensils, stainless steel kitchens, detergents, prostheses, medical appliances, metal chairs, thimbles, needles, scissors, zippers, bobby pins, fountain pens.

Occupational Exposures

Nickel mining, nickel refining, nickel electroplating, nickel alloy makers, nickel-cadmium battery workers, chemical industry, electronics and computer industry, food processing, nickel waste disposal and recycling, ceramics industry workers, duplicating machine workers, dyers, ink makers, jewelers, spark plug makers, rubber workers, plastics industry, coin manufacturers, automotive parts makers.

Signs and Symptoms

Nickel dermatitis ("nickel itch") is manifested by itching or burning causing a papular erythema of the web of the fingers, wrist and forearms. The reaction is largely allergic in nature. Acute toxicity from inhalation of nickel carbonyl: dyspnea, tachypnea, headache, insomnia, fever, cyanosis, apathy, anorexia, vomiting, diarrhea, pulmonary cancer (from nickel in tobacco smoke).

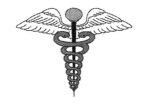

Appendix III: Monographs

> In an effort to make this work as complete as possible, we are including various monographs issued as updates following the last edition *Chronic Fatigue Unmasked.*

The Art of Healing CFS

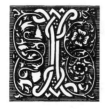

N our experience, few doctors, and even fewer patients, have an understanding of the process needed to bring the Chronic Fatigue Syndrome (CFS) patient to a state of optimum health. In this monograph we shall attempt to explain the necessary healing pattern of CFS in as simple terms as possible given the rather convoluted nature of the cure.

Most of that which follows has been presented in one or more of the books we have written on this subject in the past and yet it seems that this message has not been fully understood since questions regarding these reactions are still the most common ones posed to us by our CFS patients. So we shall attempt once again to describe the path to a healthy glandular system with all the clarity we are able to muster.

One of the main reasons that a new interpretation of this Path to Health is required is the fact that, since our exposure on the Internet, we are now seeing more patients in the later stages of CFS than we did previously. If these patients are to receive the benefit they deserve from our therapy, they must not only follow our protocol carefully, but also understand and accept the various reactions that are a natural part of their recovery.

CFS Patients as We Usually Find Them

By the time Chronic Fatigue Syndrome patients come to us, they have usually been treated for their condition for several years with little or no real improvement. Generally, they have reached a certain plateau where they are not particularly getting worse, but they certainly are not getting better. Our experience tells us that the mechanism behind this situation is usually as follows:

1. They have experienced some form of unremitting stress that has prepared the soil for full-blown CFS to manifest. Then, on top of this low-grade unremitting stress, they experienced an episode of more acute stress (accident, operation, bacterial or viral infection, death of a loved one, etc.) that pushed them "over the edge" into frank Chronic Fatigue Syndrome.

2. They eventually seek help from a local health care provider. Such help may consist of everything from reassurance and solicitation to antidepressants and cortical steroids. If they are more natural-healing oriented, they may seek Chiropractic or Naturopathic care and be placed on various nutritional supplements to build and support the affected glandular structures.

3. These measures may offer some improvement for their condition if the assault on their glandular system is not too great or if they do not have a constitutionally weak glandular system. However, in the more severe patients (those we usually see), these treatments are only band-aids and may actually make any real improvement more difficult than if they had not been employed. This is particularly true concerning the use of medically prescribed cortisone compounds.

4. Eventually the Chronic Fatigue Syndrome patient reaches a state where the body has recovered from its first stage of

exhaustion and enters Dr. Selye's "resistive" stage.[1] It is in this stage that most CFS patients come to us. In the resistive stage of CFS, the patient's body has gone into a "corrective" mode in which it is attempting to overcome the exhaustion created by the stress on the glandular system by motivating the emergency vitality reserves of the body.

In this stage, the body begins to draw upon reserve stored vitality of the glandular system. As it does, the patient feels better since the body is attempting to mimic a stable healthy condition but, with each passing day, more and more of the body's vital reserve energy is expended. Once this reserve vitality is used up, the patient will enter glandular failure and utter deep exhaustion for which the body has no mechanism to compensate.

5. The patient must realize that in the resistive stage of Chronic Fatigue Syndrome the glandular system is still in a state of weakness even though the patient may feel less exhausted than before. The feelings of strength the patient is experiencing are due to the overstimulation of his weakened glandular system by a body attempting to create homeostasis (normal balance) in them.

6. In this resistive stage, the body does all it can to respond to the needs of the patient, even though with each stimulative effort made the glandular system becomes constitutionally weaker and weaker. The deceptive feelings of patients in this stage of Chronic Fatigue Syndrome (about 80 percent of our CFS patients) are that the more they "push," the better they feel and the more they rest, the worse they feel. But, when we initiate treatment to regenerate their glandular system by enticing the body to cease its efforts at destructive overstimulation, they often discover that they feel more exhausted than before our treatment began. All we have done, however, is to have stopped

---

[1] See chart by Dr. Selye in Chapter Five, p. 91.

the artificial "high" their body was attempting to create and brought them to a status where real regeneration and a return to true vigor and vitality is eventually possible.

Since we have great empathy for all our patients, we can certainly understand their concern when, and if, they feel more exhausted than previously, following our initial treatments, but we also realize that the course of continued stimulation of an already weakened glandular system is the road to ultimate system failure and will never result in the "cure" they so ardently seek and deserve.

7. We can gain an insight into the proper and needed treatment of resistive stage Chronic Fatigue Syndrome patients by examining how the body manages the regeneration of the glandular system for normal individuals following acute infections. During an acute infective condition (say a severe case of influenza) the body goes to the "well" of stored glandular energy and utilizes all that is needed to support its needs during the stage of the disease where the body is actively fighting the invading agent. During this time, while the patient is weak (due to the fact that the body's energy is deflected away from its normal activities) he is usually alert and the body's activity is high. However, once the battle is won, and the hyperactive state of the glandular system is no longer required, a strange event occurs. The patient now usually becomes very exhausted and the temperature, that was elevated, may well drop below normal. This condition, called postviral exhaustion by the medical community, may last for several days, or even weeks, if the viral condition was severe.

This exhaustive reaction is the body's process of encouraging regeneration of the stressed glandular system following the infection and, equally important, of restoring the emergency vitality stores that were used to fight the infection. If the patient rests and gives in to this exhaustion and not force activity on the body until it has been able to fully accomplish both of these tasks, the glandular system and the body emergency stores will return to normal status in relatively short order and be ready for whatever new stress may come down the pike.

If, on the other hand, the individual does not rest until regeneration is completed (few employers are willing to give the needed sick leave once the fever has subsided) but "pushes" himself to early activity, the glandular system may well remain in a weakened state and the vitality stores never fully replaced. This scenario is one of the most common initiating causes of Chronic Fatigue Syndrome.

The Chronic Fatigue Syndrome patient, in the resistive stage of this condition, is in the same (although much more chronic and severe) state as the influenza patient who attempts to force himself back to work too soon following his infection. In both instances the body is not allowed to do its regeneration work but is, instead, forced to do the best it can with a weakened glandular system and depleted vitality stores. Unless this situation is corrected by a system of treatment that allows for full and complete regeneration, final disaster must be the end result in both instances.

What a Patient Should Expect from Our Treatment

In our early days of treating CFS, most of our patients were in the preresistive stage. That is, they came to us during the first exhaustive stage.[2] As the years went by, we began to see patients in later and later stages of Chronic Fatigue Syndrome. These patients did not respond in the same manner as our early patients did. After we initiated treatment, they began to feel more and more exhausted. At that time, we had no explanation for their increased weakness. However, we soon realized that, with treatment, they were beginning to experience the "naked" state of their unstimulated glandular system.

---

[2] See chart by Dr. Selye in Chapter Five, p. 91.

We had, in essence, begun the regeneration of their glandular system by convincing their body that it did not need to continually stimulate their glandular system, but could withdraw its efforts at such stimulation and allow the glandular system to rest and, thereby, regenerate. The result, on the patient, is similar to a "speed" junkie who suddenly has his drug removed. His built-in "crutch" has been withdrawn by the body and true regeneration has begun. It is during this stage of the Chronic Fatigue Syndrome patient's care that he most needs our Sanctuary if his condition is of any severity.

It is also during this essential stage of regeneration that the patient requires the most moral support and compassion. It is not easy for CFS patients to accept the fact that they are going through the only process that will return them to normal when they feel so tired and exhausted. On the positive side, however, they will also find that, during the regenerative treatment stage, they are much more relaxed than before and the insomnia which plagues most patients in the resistive stage, is now considerably improved, if not entirely relieved.

How Long Does the Regenerative Process Take?

The correct answer to this question is, even though it may seem a bit flippant, until the glandular system of the patient is fully regenerated. This may take from one to six months or even longer in those patients with severely depleted glandular systems.

While we attempt to treat as many of our CFS patients as possible on an outpatient basis, this is usually not completely successful with the more severe or chronic patients. In all honesty, we have, in the past, attempted to accommodate our patients and treat them as outpatients when we knew that they really required the more intensive care of our Sanctuary. We will continue to do so if the complete inpatient care is not feasible for any patient, but we do ask that all chronic Chronic

Fatigue Syndrome patients (those who have had the condition for more than a year) consider coming to our Sanctuary so they can receive the care necessary to fully regenerate their glandular system and return them to functional productivity.

Conclusion

Succinctly stated, any valid treatment of Chronic Fatigue Syndrome has to be based on the following principles and criteria:

A. The weakened glandular system must be brought back to a state of strength.

B. This cannot be accomplished except by placing the patient in a situation in which the glandular system has the needed opportunity to regenerate. Please take note of the important difference between stimulation and regeneration. To stimulate a gland may give a short term of increased activity, but further weakens an already weakened gland. To regenerate a gland is to allow that organ to regain its normal functioning by rest, specific glandular nutrition and passive modality therapy.

C. There is always a time factor involved in such regeneration. Since each Chronic Fatigue Syndrome patient is unique in his degree of glandular system exhaustion, each has his own individual schedule of regeneration.

D. Therefore, the time needed for the glandular regeneration of any individual patient is dependent on several factors:

1. The inherent quality of the patient's glandular system.

2. The severity of the original assault on the patient's glandular system.

3. The length of time that the patient has been symptomatic with CFS.

4. The extent of treatment (or lack thereof) previously received by the patient.

5. The nature and enthusiasm of the patient's cooperation.

6. The ability of the patient to access all our facilities.

It is essential that the Chronic Fatigue Syndrome patient understand the treatment principles and is willing to cooperate in his own recovery. Where lasting doubt exists concerning treatments, no total regeneration can take place.

Most Chronic Fatigue Syndrome patients we see come to us in the Resistance Phase of this condition.[3] They frequently are functioning better than the actual state of their glandular system would indicate because of an heroic attempt by the body to use its stored emergency energy to support their weakened glandular system. However, this stored energy is not being replaced and, once it becomes depleted, the CFS patient will enter a final exhaustive state for which the body cannot compensate. In this stage, few successful treatments are available and even the best of these can take years to give any substantial improvement. Therefore, every effort must be made to properly treat CFS while the patient is still in the resistive stage.

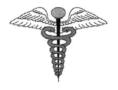

---

[3] See chart by Dr. Selye in Chapter Five, p. 91.

Life Mastery: A Protocol for CFS

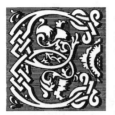 ARLY in my professional career, I had the great good fortune to be accepted as a protege of Dr. John Bastyr, a man who was, at that time, considered the wise old head of natural healing in America. Though Dr. John has now left us, he had the honor of living to see the largest Naturopathic school in the nation carry his name. Today the John Bastyr College of Naturopathic Medicine is a unit of Bastyr University in Seattle, WA.

It was this same Dr. John Bastyr who, some forty years ago, first gave me a hint about the condition that is now called Chronic Fatigue Syndrome. It was also he who introduced me to the orthostatic blood pressure test for this condition, a test just recently "rediscovered" at Johns Hopkins University.

Never having been one that could do things half way, my interest in these neglected, and often abused, patients soon became a personal crusade, one that continues to this day. Over the last forty plus years, I have discovered that Chronic Fatigue Syndrome (what I called Adrenal Syndrome for the first thirty-some years of my practice because the rest of the medical community would not even accept its existence) is one of the simplest conditions to understand and treat, but also one of the most difficult. This paradox exists because CFS can range from vague mild symptoms to near complete debilitation. While the underlying condition remains the same, its character is obviously different at these two extremes of severity. Therefore, the treatment of any one stage of CFS must be unique to that individual stage. But, I am getting ahead of myself. Let us first look and see just what we mean by Chronic Fatigue Syndrome.

What Is CFS?

In a nutshell, my long experience and, more importantly, successful treatment of CFS has convinced me that:

Chronic Fatigue Syndrome is the result of a weakening of

the glandular system (particularly the adrenal gland) of a susceptible individual as the result of long-term unremitting stress in his life.

The more susceptible the individual, the less stress and the shorter time required to create this condition. Conversely, the stronger the individual's glandular system the greater the amount of stress and the longer it must be continuously applied to manifest the condition. At one extreme of this susceptibility, we find the individual in whom CFS is triggered by the glandular changes of puberty. These individuals may well never know what real energy feels like unless they are treated by "one who knows."

On the other extreme, we have the individual who, for all practical purposes, is nearly immune to CFS, in that his glandular system is so strong that he is able to readily fend off almost any long-term stress he may encounter. Chronic Fatigue Syndrome may develop in this individual, but only following the most gigantic of personal challenges.

Four decades of research has shown that this condition is not a problem most Americans are in danger of developing unless they are exposed to very severe unremitting stress over a long period of time. My own estimate is that only from 20 to 25 percent of the general population are readily susceptible to CFS. My research has shown that, if you took a thousand average Americans and subjected them to unremitting stress for a long period of time, you might expect the following results: (1) A few individuals, those with a very strong glandular system, would show little or no effect from the stress. (2) A very large group, maybe 70 to 75 percent, would develop all the well-known symptoms of hypertensive disease (elevated blood pressure, high blood fats, etc.—leading to a susceptibility to heart attacks, strokes, etc.). (3) The remaining individuals, a smaller group than the last, but still very significant at approximately 20 or more percent of the population, would develop one or more of the various symptoms we now group under the name Chronic Fatigue Syndrome.

The reactions to unremitting stress in this last group is just the opposite from those in the group (2). When under stress, the blood pressure of those in group (3) goes down, not up. Their blood fats are rarely a problem. Not only is salt not a problem for these individuals, as it is for the majority group (3), but taken properly may well serve to make them feel better.

In discussing group (3), I am reminded of the experiments by one of the early investigators of the endocrine gland system. He removed the adrenal glands from a cat and found that when this cat was confronted by a dog it did not run or fight but simply collapsed. This is exactly the way CFS patients respond to stress. This animal experiment, and its human similarities, provide us with strong suspicions that one of the underlying causes of the symptoms of Chronic Fatigue, etc., is functional adrenal insufficiency.

As mentioned previously, there is a great variation in the degree of susceptibility to Chronic Fatigue Syndrome in this stress sensitive group. This degree of susceptibility ranges from those who would develop symptoms only under the most severe stress all the way to those who have little chance to escape Chronic Fatigue Syndrome no matter how little stress they encounter in their life. It is this latter subgroup that I have called Chronic Adrenal Syndrome individuals in some of my earlier works on this subject.

What Are the Symptoms of CFS?

As per the name given it, the most common symptom of CFS is weakness and fatigue with little or no known reason to explain it. In some phases of this condition, however, panic attacks and insomnia may well be the most prominent symptoms. It all depends on just what the body is doing to adapt at that particular point in the development of this condition.

Perhaps the most difficult pattern of symptoms for the non-CFS individual to understand about these patients is the sudden mood changes the condition can cause. Since CFS directly affects both the glandular and the nervous systems, it can bring about almost instant changes through either. A CFS patient can feel fine one moment and yet be ready to commit suicide a few minutes later. On the other hand, I have seen patients who, one day, I felt would be permanently bedridden, up and around the next day in a happy state of mind. What is happening is that these CFS patients have lost the ability to adapt or to build an internal "buffer" to the trials and tribulations we all face. Each day they walk a narrow tight rope and, if they take one misstep, they will fall into a black bottomless abyss on one side or the other.

With such quixotic mood changes, it is easy to understand why less compassionate and understanding physicians often consider these individuals to be neurotic, if not actually psychotic. It is most unfortunate, in this so-called enlightened age regarding Chronic Fatigue Syndrome, that so many doctors still consider these poor wretches to be only lazy malingerers or victims of a simple state of depression. Last night on a TV show, I saw a comedian attempting to make fun of people with what he called the "Yuppie Flu." It was a good thing that I was not in his audience or he would now have a black eye. Such ignorance! How do you think his audience would have reacted had he attempted to make jokes about diabetic or cancer patients?

What We Can Specifically Do to Help

The following protocol is particularly intended for all Chronic Fatigue Syndrome patients. It is especially designed to help the most severe of these neglected and unwanted souls. Through our past programs we have been able to return hundreds, if not thousands, of Chronic Fatigue Syndrome patients to efficient, productive lives and trust that with this new improved protocol we shall be able to help thousands more to truly live once again.

What Do We Mean by Life Mastery?

Unlike the adrenalless cat in the experiment we mentioned, our patients still have some adrenal function. The integrity of this function will vary from patient to patient, but as long as there is still some adrenal activity, it can be supported and husbanded. One of the major considerations with these patients, however, is the fact that they have very little ability to adapt quickly to the rigors often required in normal daily life. That is, the daily routine that has been designed by those from the hypertensive majority [group (2)]. We usually find hypotensive CFS patients attempting to adapt to a world made for and by another group of people. Thus, they usually go through life a square peg attempting to fit into a round hole.

Here at the Clymer Research Healing Center and Sanctuary, we have two main programs to help these patients. First, we provide, at our Sanctuary, an environment specifically designed for their adaptive abilities and, second, we have created a new protocol we call Life Mastery in which we carefully instruct these patients how to live in a world not of their own making.

In our Life Mastery program, the patient is taught how to best maximize the use of his glandular and immune systems. Unlike the hypertensive individual, the Chronic Fatigue Syndrome patient has little, or no, leeway in living his life. He must make the most efficient use of every action and activity if he is to survive in the world built by and for others. The main purpose of the Life Mastery program is to teach the Chronic Fatigue Syndrome patient how to establish this needed efficiency and effectiveness.

The Rules of Life Mastery

Rule #1

Since the CFS patient has much less vitality to expend compared to the average person: Wasted or unproductive energy expenditure must be reduced to a minimum.

Unlike the majority of the population who have the ability to bumble through life learning by trial and error, the CFS patient has little slack to do so and, if he is to survive and prosper, must learn to do things right the first time as much as possible. This takes careful instruction in Life Mastery and such instruction is the backbone of our healing care.

What we call "waste" is any unnecessary activity that is not designed to result in an improvement in the patient's basic condition. Obviously, if the patient must, and is able to, work this is a necessary activity; even though it may be a stress, it is one we must accept in many patients.

In practice, Rule #1 must be approached with reason and logic. The idea is not to make the patient a prisoner of his or her own life-style restrictions but only to reduce all activities to those that are truly to the patient's benefit on all his various functional levels. The key, as in so many things, is proper and efficient use, not nonuse or abuse.

Actually, there is no one who could not benefit from our Life Mastery program, but for the CFS-type patient it is an absolute necessity and a real life saver.

Rule #2

Since foods, and even some nutritional supplements to which the individual may have an adverse reaction, create unnecessary stress: No food, herb or supplement should be taken that does not directly contribute to an improvement of the condition.

This is actually a variation of Rule #1, something that is true of almost all the other rules that follow. Every substance that enters the body sets up a chain of events for digestion, absorption and assimilation that requires some of the body's energy. If the substance (food, vitamins, herbs, drink, etc.) takes more energy from the body than it provides, it is detrimental to the CFS patient and he will lose energy and vitality if he consumes it. This same principle applies to drugs of all kinds—prescribed or over-the-counter—whether taken by mouth or by injection. Many drugs given to CFS patients may have a seemingly beneficial short-term effect but frequently the long-term results are to the detriment of the basic CFS condition.

We are often asked for a diet to help cure CFS. Unfortunately, there is no one diet, or even type of diet, that has proven therapeutic. The diet must be individualized to each patient.

must be chosen so as to create the maximum benefit with the minimum of vitality drain.

This is usually best accomplished by a diet composed of fresh natural foods prepared in such a manner that they are easily digested so as to retain as much of their original nutrient value as possible. Also, all foods need to be combined with other foods in such a way that they impose the least amount of stress on the digestive system and are, thus, more fully assimilated.

As a part of the Life Mastery program, each individual's dietary needs will be determined and, from this evaluation, he will be taught how to choose and prepare the foods best adapted for him. While we have suggested some general dietary guidelines here, we accept as true the admonition, "One man's meat is another man's poison," so, in the long run, each CFS patient's dietary regime must be carefully adapted to his own individual requirements.

This same admonition holds true for supplements. Not only do different phases of CFS require different supplemental help, but each patient within a group invariably requires a unique supplement program as well. This, again, is a part of the Life Mastery program.

Such a supplement regime is never a fixed item. Due to the nature of CFS and its allied conditions, the needs of the patient change frequently (especially in the early stages of treatment). It is important that the physician stay on top of this situation and be ever ready to alter the supplement program if needed to meet the varying nature and needs of the CFS patient.

Rule #3

Since the glandular system of the CFS patient cannot discriminate between the various types of stress that compromise it: It is as important to prevent wasted mental and emotional energy as physical energy.

After devoting some forty years to the study and treatment of CFS, I can state, without fear of contradiction, that I have found very few cases that did not have a problem with both mental and emotional stress as well as with physical stresses. In my original books on this subject, I made the "rash" statement that one unit of mental stress was equal to two units of physical stress and one unit of emotional stress was equal to four units of physical stress. As the years have passed I have found no reason to change this conclusion or the formula itself.

Mental stress is that which might occur from an employment or occupation that involves a great deal of mental effort or concentration, but not necessarily an emotional reaction to that effort. If there is also an emotional reaction along with the mental stress, we have a combined stress assault that can become most deadly and debilitating to Chronic Fatigue Syndrome individuals.

Over the years, we have found mental and emotional stresses to be most elusive and factors that 99 percent of the physicians who treat these conditions tend to ignore. One of the main reasons for initiating our Life Mastery course is to directly address these specific stresses.

To this end, we have not only devoted a goodly part of our in-house Sanctuary program, but have also developed a correspondence program for those individuals who are not able to come to our Sanctuary at this time.

The basic principle of our program to reduce mental and emotional stress is to help the patient transmute those stresses into feelings and emotions that are constructive and productive in his nature, that is, to change hate to love, resentment to compassion, etc.

This may sound almost too good to be true but it can, and must, be accomplished if the Chronic Fatigue Syndrome patient is really to learn to live a useful and productive life. The scientific principle involved is based upon the fact that it is possible to retrain the cells of the nervous system (from the brain on down) to respond differently to stimuli than they have in the past. Our series of Life Mastery lessons, which are an integral part of this program, is the main vehicle by which the patient is taught to accomplish this most essential transformation.

Rule #4

Since, by the time we get the CFS patient, he usually has some sort of secondary immune weakness: It is essential to remove all stresses of an allergic or infective nature at the same time as the underlying Chronic Fatigue Syndrome condition is addressed.

While there is a great deal of effort to identify some specific causative agent as the culprit in Chronic Fatigue Syndrome, I do not believe that such an agent exists. We do find that, since there is abundant evidence to show that the immune system is compromised in most of these patients, they are very susceptible to the aggressive actions of various opportunistic organisms. The question here becomes one of the proverbial chicken and the egg. My experience and logic tell me that the glandular imbalance and weakness come first in most instances.

In our history of treating the CFS patient, we commonly hear the story of a patient who has been working extra hours, going short on sleep, eating mainly junk food and then, suddenly, "caught some sort of bug" and has not really felt well ever since the infection. I feel the "bug" was just the triggering mechanism for a glandular collapse that was bound to happen.

However, once the immune system is compromised and some form of opportunistic agent has "taken root," we must do all we can to assist the immune system in the elimination or shackling of this unwanted guest. In this process, we must be careful that we do not "throw out the baby with the bath water," that is, we must do all we can to see that the treatment given for the infective or allergic agent is less stressful to the patient than the agent itself.

How Do We Carry Out These Goals?

The first step in our healing efforts is to determine if our patient really has CFS and, if so, to then determine his phase or stage, so that treatment can be correctly directed. Once this is accomplished, we next begin an exhaustive examination to discover if any opportunistic organisms or other conditions are complicating the CFS condition. If these are found, appropriate treatments, in keeping with the nature of the patient's CFS phase, are instituted.

Following these efforts, special provocative noninvasive allergy tests may be advised if the patient's history leads us to believe that some form of allergy might be an inhibiting factor in his recovery. During the time that these objective examinations are being made, we will also be counseling with the patient to determine what, if any, mental or emotional support and assistance is required to assure him of a total return to the stability he desires.

Once our diagnostic work is finished, we are ready to implement our full therapeutic procedures. Due to the fact that there are certain therapies nearly all our CFS patients can use with benefit, we usually do not need to wait until all our tests are final to begin our general body regeneration efforts. However, once we have the results of our tests, we can augment our general regeneration efforts with specific therapies for the individual needs of the patient.

For patients in one of the later phases of Chronic Fatigue Syndrome, or who come to us from out of state or country, we have established our Sanctuary. This is a facility situated between our two Healing Research Centers and in easy walking distance of both. Here, the CFS patient is able to be sequestered in a world where we are able to reduce stresses to a minimum. Often the only treatment we can give at first to some of our more severe CFS patients is the stress reduction of our Sanctuary and our passive modality therapies. This combination has never failed us.

Many patients have written us stating that, while their CFS condition has improved with the care of other physicians and facilities, they eventually seemed to hit a brick wall and could go no further. Our experience has shown that the protocol outlined here, including a stay in our Sanctuary, is just what they need to break through that brick wall. We have yet to find a CFS patient who has not responded to the combination of our active and passive glandular regenerative therapy plus the required stay at our minimal-stress-environment Sanctuary.

Conclusion

The main reason our continued efforts to help CFS patients are successful is our dedication to these patients. Treating CFS is not a sideline with us; it is what we do. The vast majority of our facilities are directed to the creation and implementation of the ideal care of the CFS patient. Because of the unique nature and quixotic course of this condition, the CFS patient has many problems in his relationships with others. CFS patients are, by nature, giving individuals and when they become too weak to give, they begin to feel guilty. This sense of guilt, in turn, creates more stress which, in turn, stresses them further, worsening the condition and an unending vicious circle is created. Our Life Mastery course is designed to break this cycle of emotional pain, exhaustion and guilt by teaching these patients the rules needed to adapt their glandular system's rather unusual idiosyncracies to the outer world.

Our Life Mastery course takes into consideration all the known components of treatment that have shown promise in assisting in the correction of CFS and other allied conditions.

In fact it will help almost all known conditions that are exacerbated by any form of stress. In review, our treatment consists of:

a. Passive therapeutic modalities to help the glandular and immune systems to regenerate.

b. Carefully selected and adapted nutritional supplementation to support these two important systems.

c. Programs of counseling to assist the patient in the reduction of mental and emotional stress.

d. Specific efforts to identify and treat all allied conditions and opportunistic invaders.

e. A Sanctuary where those who require, or desire, it may

come to take advantage of a stress-free environment for their complete recovery.

Our Life Mastery course is available in three different forms:

1. A complete form in which the patient stays at our Sanctuary while being treated and instructed.

2. An outpatient form in which the patient has treatment and instruction at one of the Healing Research Centers, but lives at home.

3. A correspondence course for those patients who are not able to make it to our Healing Research Centers except, perhaps, for the diagnostic workup.

Every CFS patient, as well as those with related conditions (most auto immune conditions), can be helped to lead productive lives once again. However, to accomplish this worthy goal, every facet of their life must be taken into consideration. If problems are detected, these must be corrected if we are to be successful in our efforts to "bring back from the dead" another CFS patient. It has been our experience of the last forty years that unless the total approach, as outlined herein, is taken, there is little chance of a lasting "cure" for the more seriously affected CFS patient and so it is to these dear neglected and misunderstood individuals that our Life Mastery course is directed and dedicated.

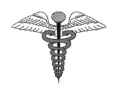

A Letter from a Friend of One Who Suffers with Chronic Fatigue Syndrome

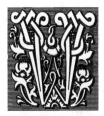E live in an age when the sensitivity toward, and compassion for, individuals who have disabilities of all types is at a high level. Unfortunately, we find that many people have a great deal of trouble extending this same understanding to those suffering with Chronic Fatigue Syndrome (CFS).

The reasons for this apathy toward the plight of these individuals are not difficult to understand. Usually the CFS patient does not look sick to the unpracticed eye. Even doctors are frequently very dubious about the validity of these patients' condition since all their test results are usually in the normal range. After all, if a doctor can't find anything wrong with them, can they really be sick? We all get tired, but we don't go around making it a lifetime avocation. Wouldn't it be best for these people to just forget about their "illness" and get back to work like the rest of us? If they are depressed, why don't they just take some Prozac® and embark on a good active exercise program? Isn't this condition just a form of "cop-out" for laziness? After all, if it is a weak adrenal, why don't they just take a cortisone drug and get it fixed up?

These are only a few of the many reasons that CFS patients have not, over the years, been treated with the respect and deference their condition warrants. The main reason for this misperception regarding CFS patients is the fact, just now being accepted by the more advanced medical researchers, that those individuals who are susceptible to CFS are not like the rest of society and, therefore, cannot be accurately judged by the criteria of the majority. They are not constructed like the rest of us and yet we expect them to react and respond as if they were. Then, when they can't do so, no matter how hard they try (and they really do try), we condemn them as being lazy, neurotic or malingerers.

The truth is that they, on the whole, are some of the most ambitious and motivated people in the world, but, unfortunately, they were born with a glandular system that does not respond to stress as does that of the majority. When most of us are under stress, our gland system will cause a rise in blood pressure and a "fight or flight" reaction. This type of manifestation is normal for most of us and continues as long as we live unless we seriously abuse ourselves.

Those individuals who are prone to CFS have an entirely different reaction. While their glands may react like those of the majority in their early years, the time soon comes when their gland system can no longer support such a normal reaction and instead of a rise in blood pressure in response to stress, the blood pressure will actually fall upon overexertion or stress. This counterreaction was discovered many decades ago by alert investigators, but was generally ignored until just recently when physicians at Johns Hopkins "rediscovered" it.

While this deviation in normal stress-related blood pressure response may not seem to be an important reaction at first consideration, it is, in essence, the key to the entire nature of the CFS person. What it demonstrates, in a loud clear language, is that the CFS patient is not a person who is likely to react to anything like the rest of us. In fact, he frequently tends to react just the opposite to the way most of us do to almost every type of human situation. Since he is not like us, does not feel or respond like us, any attempt to judge him by our standards is not only doomed to failure but usually does a great disservice to the CFS person.

If we reconsider our assessment of these CFS individuals in light of our new understanding about their inherent nature, we can now see why they cannot do as we might do and achieve the same results. If they are to survive, they must learn to manage their lives according to the nature and character of their own unique glandular makeup.

Answers to the Questions We Have Posed

The CFS patient usually does not look sick because he is not really "sick" as we generally use that term. CFS is not a sickness in the usual meaning of the word. It is, rather, a weakened condition of the glandular system (particularly the adrenal gland) that manifests its obvious symptoms only when the endocrine glands cannot send forth sufficient vitality to meet the immediate needs of the individual. The CFS patient cannot hide his condition to the practiced eye however. The eyes may well be the windows of the soul, but they are also the windows to the glandular system to those who know what to look for and who are willing to not only look, but to see. For those who are alert (and know what to look for) the CFS patient stands out in a crowd as if he had the red "A" of Hester emblazoned on his bosom.

CFS patients very frequently have normal standard blood chemistry tests. The reason for this is given above. These individuals are not sick in the ordinary sense. That is, they may well not have the kind of conditions that plague the majority of humanity, diseases for which the regular blood chemistry tests were created. There are, however, special tests available that will readily demonstrate the true nature of their condition, but these are not a usual part of the general medical workup. Why not? Because, almost all standard medical tests are wisely directed at the needs of the majority of patients. Given the medical needs-vs-cost argument so rampant today, it is only reasonable to expect this approach from the medical community. However, these neglected CFS patients do need, and deserve, a champion and it has been my pleasure to humbly serve in this capacity for over four decades now.

One of the most hurtful comments to a true CFS patient is that he is malingering. That is, that he is not really feeling as bad as he lets on and if he just would "push" himself a little more he would feel fine once again. Nothing could be further from the truth. We need to be wary of the age-old misconception that "everyone thinks and responds as we do." While in general life this concept is dubious, with CFS individuals it can lead to serious misunderstanding. CFS patients just do not react or respond like the rest of us. I know I have stated this dictum several times before, but it cannot be repeated too often, since it is the "key" to understanding and helping all CFS individuals. The world, as we know it, was built by non-CFS people. Efforts to fit CFS patients into our world is like attempting to force a square peg into a round hole. CFS patients, with proper treatment, can, and must, learn to live in a world not designed for them, but, along the way to this goal, they need the help and understanding of all those around them, who, hopefully, will never have the misfortune to learn the devastating nature of this condition from personal experience.

Drugs like Prozac® can only disguise the symptoms of the CFS patient. While there may be a place for such medication in the rare CFS patient for a short time, we generally find that all such drugs tend to worsen the CFS condition in the long run since they create a stress that further weakens the patient's glandular system.

One of the cardinal facts concerning the underlying nature of CFS is that those things that depend on the reactive ability of the body for their manifest benefit usually make CFS patients worse because they have lost much of their innate ability to react properly. This is especially true regarding exercise. That which builds the muscles and strength of the average person only further weakens the CFS patient. However, as the CFS patient is treated and the glandular system improved, a carefully monitored set of exercises can be suggested, but these need to be prescribed by a physician well versed in treating CFS patients and by no one else.

After successfully treating thousands of CFS patients, I can state one fact without the slightest fear of contradiction. They are not unproductive because they want to be. The most difficult task I have with CFS patients is getting them to rest sufficiently to allow for the needed regeneration of their glandular systems. Usually, during the course of our treatment, as a CFS patient gets even a modicum of energy, he will do all he can to make up for lost time, either at his job or at home. In this orgy of energy, he will usually continue until he completely exhausts himself. Actually the true CFS patient is one of the most ambitious individuals you will ever meet. The problem is, of course, that his glandular system, and therefore his body, cannot keep up with the activity of his mind and desires. Can you imagine a more frustrating situation? Is it any wonder that, at times, CFS patients may seem a little testy. Who can say how we might respond with a similar albatross around our neck?

Almost everyone has heard of the wonders of cortisone. If these CFS patients have an adrenal gland weakness, why not just give them cortisone and be done with it? While cortisone is a very useful drug for many things, it is only of rare help in the treatment of CFS patients.

Since these patients have a functional weakness of the adrenal gland, not a pathological one, cortisone will tend to weaken their adrenal gland further if it is used for any length of time. The normal adrenal gland excretes some forty-plus substances required by the body and cortisone is only one of these forty. When it is administered to the CFS patient, it tends to suppress the formation and distribution of the other two score substances.

How Do We Know a Person Has CFS?

In my early days of treating this condition, it was very difficult to differentiate CFS from a wide variety of other weakening conditions. We now have various new tests (such as the Adrenal Stress Index) that allow us to make a definitive diagnosis without fear of mistake. Not only do these tests tell us if an individual has CFS but, more importantly, exactly the specific stage of this condition that the patient is experiencing. Yes, CFS does meander through several stages as the glandular system, in its weakened condition, goes through various gyrations attempting to meet the needs of the CFS person. It is essential for the physician to understand the specific stage of the condition his patient is in, because the treatment must coincide with the stage or it may have an adverse effect on the patient. It is this fact that makes many physicians so reticent to treat CFS patients. There is no such thing as a standard treatment that will fit all CFS patients or even the same CFS patient at a different stage in their glandular progress. Chronic Fatigue Syndrome is not treated very successfully by those who are not willing to devote most of their healing efforts to the care of these neglected souls.

What Is the Treatment CFS Patients Need to Get Well?

Our basic treatment for CFS is threefold. First, we must do whatever is necessary to minimize the stress in the life of the CFS patient. Toward this end, the physician must always remember that stress is often not so much what happens to an individual but how he perceives that happening. Stresses can be physical, mental or emotional. Usually, physical stress is the least harmful and emotional the worst. In a severe advanced condition, the patient may even find it difficult to do the most essential daily tasks. The simple task of brushing one's teeth may create sufficient stress to force a CFS patient to rest for hours. In the most severe cases, the patient may become totally bedridden. The obvious goal of a wise physician is to control a CFS patient's stress level early on so that he does not reach these levels of severity.

Second, we search carefully for and correct any concomitant medical conditions that may be acting as unseen stresses on our patient. The CFS condition produces immune system weakness that opens the door for opportunistic organisms and adverse conditions to ravish the body. These must be tracked down and eliminated before full recovery is to be expected.

Third, the glandular system needs to be supported by passive and by active treatments to help the body regenerate both the immune and the glandular systems. This is the most important and, yet, the most difficult part of the entire therapy. This must meet the stage of the patient.

Passive treatments use those special modalities that require no effort on the part of the patient or their body to benefit. The Magnatherm is a prime example of this type of therapy. It helps organs to regenerate with no reaction needed on their part. In late stage patients, this is often the only form of therapy that can be tolerated during the beginning of their treatment.

Active treatments are those therapies that require the body or the patient to "react" to the therapy. The problem with so many CFS patients is that their body's ability to react has been deeply compromised by the condition to such a degree that such active treatments may actually place a greater stress on these patients than these therapies correct. It is up to the knowledgable physician to carefully gauge just how much active treatment, and which treatments, his patients can properly utilize at any one time. This is the true art of treating CFS and it is not to be easily or quickly learned. At our Healing Research Centers we have been doing this for nearly forty years and still find it often difficult to calculate, ahead of time, the degree of active treatment any specific patient will be able to use to his advantage.

How Long Will the Treatment Take?

By now, it should be obvious that the time needed to successfully treat a CFS patient depends entirely on the stage of the patient's condition. In the early stages, we can often have the patient productive in a few weeks. In the truly severe cases (what I call chronic CFS) it may take several months to a year or more for the recovery desired. The recovery time also greatly depends on our ability to have access to the patient. If we are able to bring the patient into our Sanctuary, where we have complete control over most of his stress quotient, we can usually have him on his feet in the shortest possible time. If we have to work so that we only get to see the patient occasionally and have no real control over his life stresses, obviously the needed improvements will be much slower in manifesting.

You were given this monograph[1] because you will be interacting with someone who has CFS or one of its many related conditions. We trust that this exploration and explanation of these really very nice and dependable people will aid you in your future relationship. When working with CFS persons, please remember that they do not react the same as you do to similar situations. When their adrenal gland has reached the end of its vitality, CFS persons will wilt like a balloon stuck with a pin and their vitality will not return until they are able to take time to rest, thus allowing for the needed regeneration of their adrenal gland. Your understanding and compassion, at times like this, will be greatly appreciated by all CFS persons.

There is much more I could write about the "care and feeding" of these very special friends of mine, but I must not let this effort get so long that you will not have the time to read it carefully. However, if you have further questions on some phase of the treatment for CFS or on the nature of a specific Chronic Fatigue Syndrome patient, feel free to call me at 1-800-779-3796 or 1-800-300-5168.

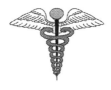

---

[1] This monograph was originally intended for Chronic Fatigue Syndrome patients to give to their employers and friends to help them to understand these individuals better.

Appendix IV: Pertinent Chapters from the 1996 Edition of *It's Only Natural*

The Electromagnetic Nature of Life: Magnatherm (Page 141)

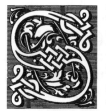INCE the beginning of man's existence on earth, he has pondered the nature of life itself. Even with all our great scientific advances, there is still no CONSENSUS on the basic nature of the life within us and other animate beings.

The most generally accepted theories are based on the chemical and/or stimulative–inhibitive theory of existence. The most we can get from most authorities is that it may be of some value to regard life as the sum total of the properties and activities of a highly organized aggregate of various chemical compounds that we call protoplasm.

Among these properties attention has been called to irritability as a diagnostic property of a living body. Upon this Herbert Spencer based his classic definition: "Life is the continuous adjustment of internal relations to external relations." Observation teaches us that this adjustment to environmental changes is possible only within narrow physiologic limits. For example, the human body can adjust itself to changes in external temperature only when these changes are very moderate.

Viewed from this angle, they hold that life is the interplay between the organism and its environment by which the organism either adjusts itself to the environment or adjusts the environment to itself.

I believe that such a definition is what our young people call a "cop-out." It tells only what life does; it doesn't tell what life is. Unfortunately, such an attitude has frequently been the nature of science since its inception. When a scientist is incapable of explaining something, he describes what he sees, makes up a few Latin or Greek names for the rest to impress us and then goes on to something else. This is particularly true in medicine, where most of the tongue-twisting disease names have nothing whatsoever to do with the cause or true nature of the disease but are only the description of its most obvious symptoms in Latin or Greek.

Some researchers haven't been satisfied with such smug descriptions of the nature of life. Some have listened to the voice of their conscience when contemplating the usual theories on the nature of life and have been able to see through the usual inane double talk couched in Latin and Greek, which all too often passes for scientific thought. They realize that much of the phenomena we encounter in living can't be explained readily by the stimulus/response theory of life as put forth by their orthodox colleagues.

Surprisingly, many of these researchers have developed concepts similar to each other, even though their work has been accomplished without knowledge of their fellow investigators. All these studies have gone beyond the chemical or mechanical basis of life and have been carried into the molecular and atomic structure of matter. From this effort first developed an electrical, then an electronic and finally a vibratory, or wave concept, of life and the activities carried out by the living subject.

Some of the most well-known researchers in this field were Dr. Georges Lakhovsky, Professor Jacques d'Arsonval (the discoverer of the meter movement that goes under his name), Dr. George W. Crile, Dr. Albert Abrams, Nicola Tesla and Ivan G. McDaniel (who advanced this theory into the psychologic, mental and spiritual spheres of human activity).

In Dr. Lakhovsky's book, *The Secret of Life*,[1] the basic theories of the vibratory nature of cellular activity are clearly and thoroughly documented. Lakhovsky hypothesized that every living bit of protoplasm emits radiations. He taught that each cell in the human body emits electromagnetic radiations similar to those from a radio station and that these radiations are of different frequencies, which act and interact, producing

---

[1] Lakhovsky, Georges. *The Secret of Life*. Rustington, Sussex, England. True Health Publishing Co., 1963.

the normal functioning of the human body. Disease, on the other hand, was held to be something that interferes or changes these radiations. To overcome disease, therefore, it is only necessary to upgrade or bring these radiations back to their normal pattern. Abrams, although approaching the subject from a different point of view, arrives at almost an identical conclusion.

Dr. George Crile, in his book *A Bipolar Theory of Living Processes*,[2] approached this subject from yet another point of view. The similarity between his conclusions and those of the other researchers in this field, however, is startling. For instance, Crile wrote, "It is clear that cellular radiation produces the electric current which operates adaptively the organism as a whole, producing memory, reason, imagination, emotion, special senses, secretions, muscular action, response to infection, normal growth and the growth of benign tumors and cancers—all of which are governed adaptively by the electrical charges that are generated by the short wave or ionizing radiation in the protoplasm."

In *Lamp of the Soul*,[3] Ivan G. McDaniel speaks of biologic wave systems that are vibratory interconnecting systems, that tend to hold a part or organ together for a specific functioning purpose. All this is based on the principle that the cell is an electromagnetic radiating entity. Concerning life on earth McDaniel says, "We may therefore picture life on earth as beginning with simple spores, or cells, which were built up by organizing wave systems when earth's conditions were suitable for life to express in that manner. As conditions changed, the fertilized genes were incorporated into the cells, bringing physical and mental growth. When a new gene and its corresponding wave system is introduced into an organism, we would expect to find the new biological wave competing with the older wave for the same cell material, and this may explain the peculiar combination of plant and animal sometimes

---

[2] Crile, George W. *A Bipolar Theory of Living Processes*. New York, Mac-Millan, 1926.
[3] McDaniel, Ivan G. *The Lamp of the Soul*. Quakertown, PA, Philosophical Publishing Co., 1942.

found in the earlier species. The balance of the activating hormone between the old and the new biological wave systems may flow back and forth until one gains control and eliminates the effect of the other by absorbing all the vitality."

I've gone into this somewhat extensive background because one must understand the basic theory of cellular vibratory activity before the different treating modalities discussed here can be properly understood. Because the nature of this work is somewhat revolutionary, I didn't want my readers to assume that any part of this theory was original, or that the treatment devices I am about to describe are based on fanciful dreams. Also, I have described the scientific character of cellular radiation because of the attitude of many in the Food and Drug Administration. This bureau, a useful watchdog at times, has among its administrators many who seem to be adherents of the chemical theories of human existence, probably stemming from their drug company-oriented and subsidized educations. Whatever the cause, they have been unsympathetic to any type of therapy that purports to function at the level of cellular electrical activity; therefore I wanted to give evidence of the soundness of the discussion to follow.

Electromagnetic Theory of Cellular Activity

The human cell, as all matter in the universe, is composed of oscillating components known as atoms, which in turn are composed of particles called protons, electrons, neutrons, and positrons, among others. All these particles are in constant movement. The movement of the electron is especially great, as it rapidly circles this central mass of the atom in various bands, or orbits. The atomic structure is analogous to our own solar system, in which the sun represents the central nuclear mass and the various planets the encircling electrons.

Any motion tends to produce pressures in a circulating fluid around a moving object, producing effects known as compression and rarefaction. The effect of such compression and rarefaction is to set up wave motions similar to the waves produced when a ball on the end of a string is whirled around one's head. The whistling sound given off by the ball is due to sound waves produced by this movement. If we make our ball move faster, if we use a smaller or larger ball, or if we add more balls, the pitch of the whistling will change. Any variation in the compression/rarefaction pattern in the air changes the nature of the sound waves emitted. Thus, matter of all kinds gives off a vibratory wave that is specific to itself. Because the combination of atoms in any matter is unique, this combination produces a wave structure that is unique, which could in turn be differentiated from all other forms of matter if we had apparatus sufficiently delicate to measure the wave or vibratory rates. Such apparatus has been constructed, though its practical usefulness is still debatable.

Because all matter is made up of atoms, the world is nothing more than a mass of structures vibrating at different frequencies and intensities. Lakhovsky and Crile expanded on this idea in their work on the living cell. Lakhovsky hypothesized that the nucleus of the living cell is so constructed that it acts as an oscillating electrical circuit, giving off not only atomic vibrations, but also waves of electromagnetic origin, similar to those generated by a radio or TV station.

Owing to the minute dimensions of the cells, the frequency of these waves is very high. He stated that the electromagnetic waves given off by the various organs are separate and distinctive, and it is the nature of these waves that enables the differentiation of fetal tissues. Each specific gene in the fertilizing cells has a characteristic wave pattern, and as growth and maturity take place, this electromagnetic pattern is gradually developed until the organ and/or personality trait is completed, somewhat like a tape-recorded program that is broadcast over the ether from a radio station.

Not only is growth under the control of these electromagnetic wave patterns, but also tissue repair. Therefore, as long as the vibratory rates in the cells remain normal, there should be no disease. If, however, these electromagnetic waves are altered, the cellular structure and its basic functioning must then subtly change and disease, of one form or another, can begin in the system. This state Lakhovsky used to refer to as oscillatory disequilibrium. Many factors can produce this oscillatory disequilibrium and it was experimentally shown by Lakhovsky, and others, that the disease-producing effects of poor diet, bacterial invasions, overindulgence in alcohol or other toxic substances, stress, anxiety, lack of sleep and similar assaults on the system can be shown to produce their effects by producing oscillatory disequilibrium.

Lakhovsky believed that what we know as infection was but a vying of the various electromagnetic oscillatory rates between the human cell and the bacterium for dominance. He theorized that the electromagnetic wave structure of the pathologic bacterium tends to interfere with the normal wave patterns of the infected organ or part and that if the body is successful in overcoming the infection, it indicates that the body's wave mechanism is sufficiently powerful to overcome that of the bacterium. If the opposite is the case, it is a sign that the bacterial vibratory patterns are sufficient to so disorient those of the body that the body cells can't function as a unit any longer and that death must ensue.

The work of these men is highly documented and very extensive. Although books on this specific matter haven't been published recently, there have been a couple of very interesting correlated researches. One is entitled *The Secret Life of Plants* by Peter Tompkins and Christopher Bird,[4] in which the authors describe the various effects of human thought waves and emotions on plant structure. They discuss experiments showing that plants respond very adversely to human anger, hatred and condemnation. If these emotions are only feigned, there is no response whatsoever on the part of the plant. In this fascinating and authoritative work, we find further support for the vibratory theory of cellular life. To me these experiments show that the electromagnetic wave energy put out by human feelings and emotions can radiate for some distance, affecting the vibratory structures of other living organisms.

---

[4] Tomkins, Peter, and Bird, Christopher. *The Secret Life of Plants.* New York, Harper & Row, 1973.

That feigned hatred and anger had no effect on these plants shows that it is neither the sound nor the fury that produces these effects, but the effect of electromagnetic vibrations produced only by the factual and not contrived emotions.

A new type of photography called Kirlian photography has been used recently to demonstrate strange emanations that come from living matter, both animal and plant. These emanations seem to me to be a visualization of the electromagnetic waves that are a part of all living structures.

Therapeutic Devices Based on These Principles

Because of the complicated nature of this subject, I suggest you read and even re-read the previous section carefully before attempting to understand the following therapies.

In considering the following therapeutic devices, two questions must be asked. First, is the theory on which the modality is based sound? Second, is the specific instrument capable of delivering the benefits of the espoused theoretical method? Specifically we are asking, "Is the cellular electromagnetic wave principle of health and disease practical and does the instrument we're using perform according to the theory and to the benefit of the patients?"

My own experience in healing has constantly confirmed the validity of the electromagnetic theory of life. Whether all the specific details described by Crile, Abrams and Lakhovsky are correct doesn't particularly interest me. It isn't essential to know exactly how these wave structures are produced or specifically interact to help a patient. Future research may somewhat modify exact findings of the early work done on this subject, but I'd be surprised if future investigation were able to invalidate the fundamental hypothesis involved. Therefore, in my own mind, treatment by electromagnetic means resolves itself down to one fundamental question. Does the instrument I am using help to normalize the electromagnetic structures of the body and to overcome the oscillatory disequilibrium, which we call disease?

Abrams' Radionic Treating Devices
and the Depolar Ray

Abrams, in his work on cellular radiation, developed two types of instruments to test his theoretical work. One was a diagnostic instrument designed to detect and classify the normal electromagnetic vibrations of tissues and of the different disease entities in the body. Due to lack of sufficiently sensitive detectors, this instrument could function only through the use of the human nerve reflex and thus its true scientific nature was difficult to verify, since the effectiveness varied with each operator. Such diagnostic instruments were tested at our Center in years past but the results were not consistent. Attempts are now being made to utilize new sensitive electronic means to determine the electromagnetic wave structures of the different organs and tissues. Until these attempts are successful, we feel, this piece of apparatus must remain only a curiosity.

The other type of instrument produced by Abrams was for treating and it used very low-power oscillating currents to produce electromagnetic waves similar to those of the human cells. The last machines of this sort, to my knowledge, were produced by the now defunct Electro-medical Company of San Francisco, headed by Fred Hart. These instruments produced various wavelengths to treat different conditions; in some, these wavelengths were applied one after the other in succession to the treating organs. This last pattern was similar to a circuit known as the Knight circuit, which was somewhat similar to Lakhovsky's multiple wave oscillator, though his instrument was based on the spark-gap principle rather than on the wave production of the triode tube used in the Knight circuit.

The energy from the Abrams machines was applied by a variety of electrodes, generally four, which were placed over various parts of the body to produce the desired effects in specific diseases. These treating machines flourished for a time in the 30's and 40's, but today, it is our understanding that they are being produced only in England for the home market.

The Fred Hart Company also produced an instrument called the Depolar Ray, which wasn't much more than a large coil of copper wire through which an alternating electrical current circulated. The basic circuit was identical to that of a "degaussing agent," an instrument used to demagnetize objects inadvertently magnetized. In the opinion of the Fred Hart Company, this alternating electromagnetic unit helped overcome problems present in congested tissue. It was originally recommended for a variety of athletic injuries, though I find the usual ice pack treatment superior. The Depolar Ray did have a valid use, however, in the benign prostatic enlargements of middle-aged men and in simple cases of hemorrhoids.

There were other types of machines based on the Abrams theories, but in general they were all variations of those just described. I know of none manufactured today in our country and more research and scientific evaluation is needed before this type of instrument is manufactured in the United States again.

The Diapulse and Magnatherm

Some time after the work of Abrams, Lakhovsky and Crile, Dr. Goldberg of New York City observed what he considered unusual effects on patients under treatment with orthodox diathermy apparatus. The diathermy machine uses a form of electromagnetic energy to radiate heat deep into the tissues. As the electromagnetic energy from the diathermy machine passes through the tissues of the body, a combination effect of hysteresis and eddy currents is produced causing thermal activity in the tissues proportional to their density and the magnitude of the electromagnetic wave. In other words, as the diathermy wave passes through the body, a sort of electrical friction is set up in the denser tissues that produces heat. The stronger the wave put through the body, the greater the friction formed and the greater the heat produced.

Dr. Goldberg detected benefits that his patients attributed to the diathermy treatment he was giving that couldn't be accounted for from the use of internal heat alone. Goldberg eventually assumed that another form of energy besides heat was imparted to the tissues by the electromagnetic wave of the diathermy machine. Further investigation led him to believe that the amplitude (strength) of the electromagnetic wave in the standard diathermy was too weak for the investigation he had in mind, so, to further examine his new effect, he had built a machine that had a much greater power than those then available. Unfortunately, the increased strength of the electromagnetic wave also increased the heat in the tissues. Because this heat was already at the maximum allowable without injuring the patient in the standard machine, it was necessary for Goldberg to find a way of increasing the strength of the electromagnetic energy without increasing the heat. To do this, he designed a machine that later became known as the Diapulse machine. The electromagnetic waves in this instrument were pulsed instead of constant. Because of this pulsing, heat did not build up in the tissues; thus, a much greater electromagnetic force could be applied than before. Goldberg could thus concentrate on the pure electromagnetic effects of the diathermy energy and his results were published in many professional journals.

The Diapulse machine was eventually produced commercially as an auxiliary aid in many diseases. It was used in many hospitals and by physicians of all the health professions. It was originally produced by Sperry Remington Rand Company and later by the Diapulse Company of America, which claimed it was useful in approximately 150 conditions. The FDA took the company to court to see if it could prove these claims. The final decision of the court was that the company could prove approximately half the claims, but the court didn't think the other half were adequately proven and they therefore could not be listed in the company's literature. Later, the FDA thought the company was still making claims that hadn't been substantiated and sought and obtained an order stopping the interstate sale of the machines.

A later decision by an FDA administrator (not a court of law as we understand it) stated that the machines, in his opinion, were worthless, and he therefore ordered their destruction or confiscation. The Clymer Health Clinic was using five Diapulse machines at this time and we believed that such a completely arbitrary and unlawful decision was entirely counter to our Constitutional rights and so we did what we could to prevent confiscation and destruction of our machines. However, it is usually impossible to fight government agencies over such confiscation, and finally all our Diapulse machines were subsequently unceremoniously destroyed. (This was the status of this matter when I wrote the first edition of this book. However, in the ensuing years the Diapulse Corporation took the government to court and finally won their case. They are now allowed to sell the Diapulse once again. Now that it was determined that the FDA had destroyed tens of thousands of dollars of our Clinic's equipment without legal cause, you might think that the government would be forced to reimburse us for the loss. That did not happen. We did not even get a "We're sorry.")

A pulsed electromagnetic generator such as the Diapulse is basically little different from the orthodox diathermy machine. If the pulses are fast enough and the power great enough, it will produce tissue heat similar to that encountered in ordinary diathermy. Therefore, it would be possible for a manufacturer to produce an instrument based on the principles of the Diapulse that could put out sufficient heat energy to function as a diathermy machine. If such a machine were produced without any claims other than those made for normal short-wave diathermy, it should not rouse the ire of the FDA.

The International Medical Electronics Company of Kansas City has produced such an instrument—the Magnatherm. Besides being a much more sophisticated instrument than the original Diapulse, the Magnatherm has also been especially helpful in our busy Centers because each unit has two separate treating heads, rather than the single one on the Diapulse. Because of this, we are able to treat our patients in half the time required for a Diapulse treatment. The Magnatherm is truly a space-age instrument. Its controls are all digital readout modular units and it even has a built-in oscilloscope so that the rate and amplitude of the wave being administered can be visually analyzed. We have several of these instruments in heavy use at both the Woodlands Medical Research Center and the Clymer Healing Research Center, and as far as I know, we are the only establishment with such an array anywhere in the country.

The use of the Diapulse, and now the Magnatherm, has been one of the backbones of the healing methods used at the Centers. Our patients well know the high regard we have for these instruments. However, it is not the Diapulse, Magnatherm or any other such instrument that makes the patient well. These instruments are but the tools of our physicians. The tool doesn't produce the final product; only the skill of the physician can do that. We could perform our cures without the Diapulse or Magnatherm, but it would be a slower and more arduous task. These machines have proven to be fine, but not indispensable, tools.

What the Magnatherm Does[5]

The electromagnetic wave pulses produced by the Magnatherm machine are used in our Centers to regenerate various organs or systems of the body directly at the cellular level. In acute conditions—those of an infectious or an inflammatory nature—the energy is used to hasten and support the body's reactive ability. In combination with other forms of natural treatment, this therapy has proven most efficacious. Experience has shown me that when properly used the Mag-

---

[5] This discussion is not based on generally accepted medical opinion. Anything I say here concerning the Magnatherm must he taken as my own opinion, arrived at from my own extensive clinical work with this method of therapy and I don't want to imply that the manufacturer of the Magnatherm in any way substantiates my opinions or conclusions.

natherm activates the reticuloendothelial system of the body, thereby hastening healing in acute disorders.

Treatment of Chronic Diseases.

It is in chronic conditions that the Magnatherm plays its major role at our Centers; in these conditions, natural therapy easily outshines its competition. To understand the reason for this success, one must first understand the nature of a chronic condition.

All acute conditions are self-limiting in that the patient either recovers and returns to his normal state, or he dies. Colds, flu, boils and pneumonia are all examples of such acute conditions.

In chronic conditions, the healing process of the body is not sufficient to cast off the offending problem, nor is the afflicting ailment strong enough or of such a nature as to destroy the vital functions of the body. We thus have a stalemate in which neither the disease nor the body defenses conquer one another. The patient thus continues to suffer until he either dies or by some means the body is finally able to overcome the disease.

Orthodox medical science has been relatively successful in the last fifty to sixty years in overcoming many acute disorders. They have, however, made little headway in dispelling chronic disease. Although some of the symptoms of these disorders may be relieved by drugs, at least temporarily, little curative help is offered for these increasingly common disorders.

The usual chronic condition must be overcome from within, not from without. The general therapeutic method most useful to us at our Centers is that which stimulates and revitalizes the body repair mechanisms so that this innate system can overcome the chronic ailment. To do this, we generally apply the following five techniques:

> 1. All known toxic substances are removed from the patient's internal and external environment. For instance, if a patient is working, we check his job environment for any form of

poisonous or toxic substances he may be breathing, ingesting or in any way contacting during his employment. His foods are also carefully selected to reduce additives and pesticide residues. His home environment is investigated to find and correct any factors that may be causing toxic reactions.

2. The patient is placed on a diet carefully adapted to him with which we hope to supply a good balance of the elements generally needed and an abundance of the elements particularly important to his specific disorder.

3. Every effort is made to establish a constructive, optimistic mental and emotional attitude to prevent the adverse effects of antagonistic vibrations that result from negative and destructive emotions .

4. Specific nutrient substances designed to act as builders of normal cell functioning are prescribed. These are carefully chosen after tests indicate the special needs of the patient.

5. Electromagnetic treatments are given to mildly stimulate the parts of the system that have become sluggish and inactive and that thereby may have enhanced the disease. In regard to this last technique, one may consider the person with a chronic ailment as someone in whom there is disorder and general sluggishness in some of the organ structures. If we can mildly stimulate these organs to aid in their regeneration, we can gradually direct their activity toward more normal function. To accomplish this fully, however, it is usually necessary to see that our first four techniques of the treatment of chronic disorders are also met.

In our own Clinic, we use electromagnetic energy in chronic disorders in both a specific and a general fashion. When we are striving for a general encouragement and regeneration of glandular and body function, we treat the liver, spleen, pancreas and adrenals. Where some specific organ is involved other than the kidneys, which will receive the electromagnetic radiation on the adrenal setting, a separate setting is also made on this part. For more specific treatment, the Magnatherm may be placed directly over the offending part, such as the knee or hips in osteoarthritis, or over the face in sinusitis.

Great care must be used in the beginning treatment of chronic cases. An old professor from medical school used to say, "You can't take these old chronic cases and try to push them to health. You must take them by the hand, and very gently lead them to health." His words have repeatedly come to mind over the years and without exception his advice has proven sound. The worse a case is, the gentler we must proceed.

The electromagnetic energy of the Magnatherm, or of the regular diathermy machine, has a potent stimulating effect on cellular activity and must be carefully used if the desired result is to be obtained. Almost any form of electromagnetic or vibratory therapy can have vastly different effects on the treated part, depending on its intensity, character and the length of time applied. For instance, if we take an electromagnetic wave and apply it at a low rate and intensity for a reasonably short time, we can produce a relaxing effect on a nerve. If we take this same electromagnetic energy, increase its frequency, or increase its strength or time, that same nerve may be stimulated. If we continue to increase the frequency amplitude and time, it is eventually possible to reach a point at which the nerve is destroyed. This is done, for instance, when the short-wave diathermy is used as a cautery unit. It is easy to see why I have stressed the physician's skill and not the machine's ability in overcoming disease. If a nerve needs to be relaxed but the practitioner operates his instrument so that a stimulative treatment is given, the patient will certainly not exhibit the desired effect. On the other hand, if a relaxing treatment is given in chronic ailments where a stimulative effect is needed to start body healing, the patient may feel somewhat better for a short time but his condition never will be structurally improved. The competent therapist must use his machines as a musician plays his instrument. He must be able to evoke in the cells and organs of the patient the exact effect needed at the time of treatment.

Almost any form of body dysfunction can be helped by a careful and judicious use of the electromagnetic force. It is really not a mysterious treating method but simply a way to produce on specific organs or other parts of the system relaxing or stimulative effects needed at that point in the progress of the disorder. This is no more irrational or mystical than the medical practitioner who gives a diuretic to stimulate the kidneys, digitalis to stimulate the heart or belladonna to inhibit alimentary canal muscles. One is a chemical stimulation–inhibition method; the other is electromagnetic. It is our experience that the electromagnetic method is somewhat weaker, but much safer and without the side effects all too common to chemotherapy.

In many of the disorders for which we use electromagnetic therapy, there are no generally recognized acceptable chemical alternatives. When the disease is of long duration, the treatment may seem to be overly long, leading some patients to complain that while natural methods are safe, they take longer than orthodox medical methods. Actually, the opposite is true. Because most medical treatment of chronic disorders with drugs is only palliative (symptoms are controlled, but no cure takes place), little time is involved, but if we attempt to cure, much time and effort must be expended. The true cure of a chronic disease is effected more rapidly through natural therapy than by any other means.

In summary, many accomplished physicians and scientists believe the cells of the body can produce and are affected by specific electromagnetic waves. Methods have been developed to measure and categorize these waves in both sickness and disease, but there is as yet no conclusive scientific evidence that these methods are entirely accurate or repeatable. Many treating modalities have been developed to make use of changing the disease wave forms into healthy tissue wave forms by electromagnetic means. Owing to the nature of the machines and of the diseases they purport to treat, it is difficult to assess these devices on an impartial, scientific basis. We have sufficient interest in several, however, to use them in research projects at our Clinic. The machines we have in daily use are generally available to the medical profession and are fully authorized by the FDA. It is the manner in which we use these machines that produces our desired effect and not some mysterious characteristic of the instrument itself.

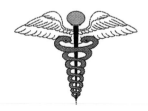

Miracle Healing with Photons (Page 107)

 NE of the latest healing advances at our Centers is a miniature marvel known as the MicroLight 830 low level laser. This unit is at the time this is being written still in its efficacy investigation stage, though I expect that by the time you read this it will be fully approved by the FDA. At this time we are a part of the investigational team assessing the therapeutic advantages of this treatment. Before we give you some of our own experience with this unit, which I affectionately call "the world's most expensive flashlight," we want you to hear from Dr. David G. Williams who had an opportunity to evaluate the MicroLight 830 before us.

The nature of this therapy and the various conditions that it is designed to treat are discussed in the following articles that first appeared in the newsletter, *Alternatives*, by Dr. David G. Williams.

"If you've ever watched an episode of the old science fiction television show Star Trek, or its newer spin-off, Star Trek, The Next Generation, you'll undoubtedly remember how simple and quickly health problems were eliminated.

"Regardless of the problem, the futuristic doctors treated each patient by simply holding a small device directly over the afflicted area. I'm not sure if the little playing-card sized device emitted some kind of gas, electromagnetic waves, or what. I just know the patient quickly got well and there was never any cutting, bleeding or removal of organs or tissue. Hey, it was just a television program. Nobody could actually develop such a device. That's what I thought, anyway, until a couple of months ago.

"For the last several months, I've been investigating a small flashlight-looking device that will probably revolutionize certain segments of health care as we know them today. A small company near Houston, Texas has developed a portable, infrared, low energy cold laser device that has demonstrated remarkable healing powers. The unit was imported by Lasermedics of Stafford, TX.

"Lasers have been around for quite some time now. In the medical field surgeons have been using them to cut, burn and vaporize unwanted tissue. Dentists are starting to use lasers instead of mechanical drills. All of these that create enough heat to burn or vaporize tissue are all high energy lasers or what is referred to as High Reactive-Level Laser Therapy (HLLT).

"Lasermedics' unit is different. It doesn't cut, burn or vaporize tissue. It falls under the category of Low Reactive-Level Laser Therapy (LLLT). A little technical background will help you better understand the unique healing ability of LLLT.

"Although I think the following information concerning light is one of the most exciting and useful health topics today, if you're not into details you can skip the next few paragraphs. If you stick with me I promise not to get too technical (When I do I usually end up getting more confused than anybody else).

"Most of us have a pretty poor understanding of light. Since it's something we can't touch or feel we don't give it much thought. All light is actually electromagnetic waves. The color of the light or whether we even see it or not depends on the length of the wave or wavelength. Any light with a wavelength between 400 nanometers (nm) and 700 nm is visible to the human eye. This is called the visual spectrum. (Nanometers, by the way aren't very long. A meter is 39.37 inches, or a little over a yard. A nanometer is one-billionth of a meter!)

"Generally speaking, the smaller the wavelength the greater its ability to penetrate tissue. Ultraviolet rays, x rays, gamma and cosmic rays all fall below visible light on the electromagnetic spectrum. But infrared rays, microwaves, television, FM and AM radio waves have much longer wavelengths.

"What most people don't understand is that light and all electromagnetic energy travels as bundles of energy called photons. (This is where things start to get a little difficult.)

"If you recall anything from your high school chemistry class you may remember that the center or nucleus of an atom contains neutrons and protons. The nucleus is surrounded by electrons moving in specific orbits. Energy in the form of photons is released when the electrons change orbits. It is these weightless bundles of energy called photons that trigger biological changes within the body.

"While random photons from ordinary light sources are constantly bombarding the surface of our skin, lasers have the ability to 'concentrate' these photons. Photons from ordinary light are emitted in all different directions. In contrast most of the photons emitted from a laser are in perfect order and follow the same path. The effects of the energy released from a laser depend on several factors. The wavelength and the wattage output of the laser are two of these factors.

"Some high energy lasers are absorbed by water within the skin, making their penetration very shallow. Others will penetrate several hundredths of an inch and vaporize any tissue in their path. And low energy laser devices are designed to penetrate deep within tissues (by utilizing a different wavelength) without causing any heat or tissue damage (by operating at very low power settings).

"Lasermedics' device operates at 830 nanometers and at the low energy output of only 30 milliwatts. This allows the photons to penetrate over an inch deep (3 centimeters) without any danger of tissue damage or destruction. If you've stayed with me so far, you're probably wondering: 'Who cares? What good are these worthless little bags of energy called photons anyway?'

The Magic of Photons

"All life on this planet is dependent upon light energy (photons) derived from the sun. The sun's energy is first captured when the chlorophyll molecules in plants absorb photons. This energy is then used in the process of photosynthesis to create glucose and oxygen.

"Through the consumption of plants, animals (this includes all humans, not just wild apes, wildebeests and your in-laws) are able to release the energy stored in glucose.

"We also receive energy directly from the sun, independent of our food supply. And even though the amount we receive is far less than that which comes from food, it is essential for good health.

"The sun's photons, which strike the skin directly, convert a form of cholesterol into vitamin D. Studies have shown that vitamin D deficiencies lead to osteoporosis and result in increased fractures of the hip and spine. Dr. Holik of Tufts University found that 30% of the elderly who experience hip fractures are deficient in vitamin D. And 50% of those evaluated in New England nursing homes were deficient in vitamin D during the winter months.

"Low levels of vitamin D have also been linked to increased rates of both breast and colon cancer (*Med Trib* 89;30:(30)1).

"Photons also enter the body through the eye. These are absorbed by several different light-sensitive chemicals like rhodopsin. Rhodopsin transfers these power bundles to the crucial little energy factories inside cells called mitochondria. Through an intricate pathway this energy is transferred to the pineal gland—a small pine cone shaped structure located exactly in the center of the head.

"The pineal gland is the 'master gland' of the body. Based on both the amount of light energy absorbed by the body and the particular cyclic pattern of the Earth's magnetic field, the pineal functions as our biological clock and regulates the operations of all the other glands in the body. We now know it controls other glands by releasing dozens of regulating chemical substances plus several major neuro-hormones like dopamine, melatonin and serotonin. Understandably, an imbalance in the amount and intensity of light energy reaching the body can lead to disastrous effects.

What Photons Do Inside the Body

"Before photons (light energy) can produce any effect they must be absorbed into the body. Then, regardless of how they were absorbed, three events can take place when their energy is released.

> "1. Heat can be generated. The more energy liberated, the higher our body temperature becomes. Any increase in activity, such as exercise, requires the release of additional energy which warms the body. (On the other hand, drinking beer while watching television conserves energy, but it makes your feet get cold.)

> "2. Another photon with less energy can be released. Our bodies aren't 100% efficient in their use of energy (no living organisms are). As such, some of the energy escapes. This leakage of energy is continuous and contributes to the energy field that surrounds all living organisms. This energy field has also been referred to as the aura.

> "3. Photons can trigger a long list of cellular changes which fall under the heading of photobiostimulation. The ability to place these photons exactly where they're needed and elicit these cellular changes will make laser therapy one of the most advanced forms of healing ever discovered.

"I need to make one thing clear before I continue. Keep in mind that whenever I mention laser therapy (or more precisely Low Reactive-Level Laser Therapy or LLLT), it's actually photons I'm talking about. Lasers are simply tools that create photons. Next time you see your doctor and mention you've become interested in photon therapy he or she will probably have no idea what you're talking about. On the other hand, while most doctors don't know about LLLT, they have heard of lasers.

"When I first started checking into LLLT, I was very skeptical. From the reports I was receiving it appeared to cure almost everything. And it's been my experience that when a therapy or product reportedly cures everything, it generally cures nothing. LLLT is a noted exception.

"From first hand experience, I can tell you LLLT is a miraculous healing tool that on the surface seems contradictory. It can alleviate the sensation of pain, but it can also bring back a sense of feeling in areas that have gone numb. It can remove overgrown scar tissue or it can stimulate tissue growth. It can remove excess pigment, but it also restores pigment in areas where needed. It can activate healing components within the immune system, but also decrease the body's sometimes harmful inflammation response. The beauty of LLLT is that its photons normalize tissue. Photons do this by activating enzymes.

"Enzymes are molecules that speed up the chemical reactions among other substances without itself being destroyed or used up in the process. By directly triggering enzymes the power of photons is multiplied by thousands through a domino-type effect. One photon can activate a single enzyme which in turn triggers a chemical reaction, which triggers another and another, etc.

"And with LLLT there have been no adverse side-effects noted. It apparently has no effect on normal tissue. It seems to act much like a nutrient. Photons will only be absorbed by the cells that need help. If a cell is functioning normally, no benefit will be observed from LLLT.

Specific Conditions Being Treated

"The full FDA approval process for Lasermedics' MicroLight 830 is expected to be completed in the near future. Safety trials have already been completed and the LLLT has been found to have no adverse effects. Selected doctors around the country are now allowed to use these units for treatment to determine the breadth of their effectiveness. These trials are under an investigative license from the FDA. If you are interested in this treatment contact one of these physicians to see if your problem falls into the parameters of this program. (We at the Healing Research Centers are now an official investigator for this therapy.)

"I have personally had the opportunity to use Lasermedics' portable laser unit, the MicroLight 830, for several weeks. I have seen chronic arthritic joint pain (duration of three years) disappear after one 3-minute treatment period. The same results have been achieved with shoulder, neck, knee and lower back pain.

"I have also conducted interviews with several of the doctors who have been testing these units in their practices for the last year or so. Each of the doctors I've spoken with had nothing but the most glowing reports for LLLT.

"Dentists have used the instrument for dry socket problems, gum disease and temporal mandibular joint (TMJ) disorders. Others have used it on keloids and scar tissue, torn knee cartilage, 2nd and 3rd degree burns, surgical and open wounds, damaged nerves, headaches, sinus problems, strains, sprains and athletic injuries.

"One of the fastest growing complaints in this country today, carpal tunnel syndrome (CTS), responds to the laser as well. CTS is caused by repetitive motion and trauma to the median nerve passing through the wrist. Assembly line workers are particularly prone to the problem. The automotive giant General Motors has found that 25% of its workers' compensation cost is from repetitive stress injuries like CTS. The standard medical treatment for CTS is still surgery, which has a dismal success rate of less than 10%. Dr. Wayne Good, the plant physician at General Motors' Flint Assembly, has treated close to 600 patients with LLLT and achieved positive results in over 70% of the patients. He is in the process of submitting his results for publication as further studies continue.

"Photobiotherapy will become one of the premiere healing tools of our future. It will eliminate the need for many of today's common surgical procedures. I can see the day when every household in this country will have an LLLT unit on hand. When used properly, it is a safe, effective, natural therapy for a wide variety of health problems. Until this happens I wanted you to be aware of an extremely effective therapy that, in many cases, could very well eliminate the necessity of surgery and the dangers associated with it.

"Photobiotherapy is nothing new. It is as old as the sun itself. Harnessing and refining this therapy through the use of 'tuned' lasers is new, and can enhance, rather than oppose, the body's own innate healing powers."

The Invisible Healing Light

"About a year and a half ago, I discovered a therapy that I considered to be a real breakthrough in natural healing: Low Reactive-Level Laser Therapy (LLLT). Based on research at that time, I was surprised that the national media hadn't picked up on the story and alerted the public. Even more surprising is the fact that LLLT still remains practically unknown among health professionals, despite continuing evidence of its effectiveness in a wide range of health problems. Numerous readers have reported getting excellent results using LLLT and hundreds of others have been asking for an update. I can tell you, since I last reported, a lot has been happening with LLLT.

"In that earlier report, I thought the FDA would quickly approve the use and sale of the MicroLight 830, the laser unit being tested and manufactured by Lasermedics. Although the FDA has approved its use, they haven't yet given the manufacturer the go ahead to market it freely. Let me share some of the latest research involving this unique apparatus.

"I originally referred to LLLT as Star Trek medicine. This was a reference to the almost magical healing properties of a small, playing-card sized device used on the television show Star Trek. By simply holding this device over a wound or injured body part, the patient would experience almost immediate healing. The more we learn about LLLT the more it seems to work like the Star Trek device.

"I'm not going to go through the detailed explanation of exactly what LLLT is or how it appears to work, since I covered that earlier. Suffice it to say that LLLT involves a device that focuses light energy in the form of photons. It delivers them to cells and organs over an inch or so below the skin without any tissue damage whatsoever. These photons have the unique ability to stimulate healing in damaged cells.

An Effective Treatment for Carpal Tunnel Syndrome

"Much of the original work with LLLT involved its usefulness in treating the condition called carpal tunnel syndrome (CTS). CTS is a condition involving the inflammation of the median nerve in the wrist. It is a type of repetitive motion injury. In other words, certain wrist movements that are performed over and over can irritate the tendons and nerves that pass through the bony tunnel of the wrist. Once the nerve becomes inflamed, symptoms like pain, numbness, tingling or a complete loss of feeling in the fingers, hand and arm are not uncommon.

"CTS is just one of many problems low reactive-level laser therapy (LLLT) treats effectively. I've seen it eliminate chronic muscle and joint pain in a matter of minutes. It can dramatically speed up the healing of wounds, strains, sprains, burns, athletic injuries, headaches, chronic skin ulcers and gum disease. Dentists are using the instrument to treat dry socket and temporal mandibular joint (TMJ) disorders. Researchers at St. Joseph Hospital in Houston, Texas, have even used the laser unit to treat Peyronie's disease.

New Hope for Peyronie's Disease

"Peyronie's disease is an inflammatory reaction, accompanied by the formation of hard fibrous tissue, that occurs in the penis. It results in painful erections and often times, a severe distortion of the penis. Standard medical therapies like surgery, or steroid or hormone injections, are generally unsuccessful. When treated with LLLT, however, eight of the eleven patients in a recent study showed significant improvement. The patients were only treated for a period of five weeks. Following that, many of the patients' problems began to return. Considering the nature of the problem, it might be necessary to continue the treatment for longer periods of time. The fact that any improvement at all was achieved is in itself remarkable. I don't know of any other therapy that has shown such positive results in that high of a percentage of Peyronie's patients.

"Studies are also underway by members of the Harvard University orthopedic department at Massachusetts General Hospital to determine the effects of LLLT on damaged cartilage cells. Early information indicates that LLLT appears to stimulate the regeneration of cartilage cells. Currently, tests are being conducted in vitro, using cartilage cells from cattle. In the next four to six months, these researchers hope to be conducting those same tests involving human cells. If the preliminary results are any indication of what will happen in human cells, LLLT could revolutionize the way arthritis is treated. The ability to regenerate cartilage would be an unparalleled medical breakthrough. Rest assured, I'll keep you up to date as we receive additional information.

"Using a special dental attachment on the laser, researchers at the famous Beckman Laser Institute, in California, have been able to prevent mucositis in radiation-treated cancer patients. Dr. Petra Wildersmith, who heads the study, will be reporting the results early next year. Laser therapy was given to twelve patients prior to their undergoing radiation therapy to the head and neck area. In all but two patients, the therapy prevented the patients from developing mucositis. Mucositis is a painful, severe inflammation of the membranes lining the mouth and throat. The problem which stems from the radiation therapy interferes with the patient's ability to eat or drink. The discovery that laser therapy can prevent the problem will be a godsend to thousands of cancer patients worldwide.

Lasers and Human Energy Fields

"In my first report, I gave a pretty detailed explanation of how light energy, in the form of energy packets called photons, promotes healing in the body. The ideas I presented have been well researched and documented; however, the idea that an invisible light can promote healing still mystifies most people. This is especially true in the Western cultures.

"In the Far East, it is common knowledge that living cells emit a form of energy or life force. For hundreds of years, acupuncturists have treated all kinds of diseases by balancing and harmonizing this energy. Many Westerners, however, continued to doubt the existence of this so-called 'Life force' until the 1960's, when newer technology enabled researchers to demonstrate that living cells emit coherent light energy called Biophotons. (Popp FA, Electromagnetic Bio-Information. Baltimore, MD: Urban and Schwarzenberg: 1989.)

"When a group of cells are functioning in harmony, they emit biophotons (light energy) at the same wavelength and rhythm. When there is damage or disease, this harmony is lost. This phenomenon has been observed and recorded by individuals 'sensitive' to these subtle energies throughout history.

"These biophotons or packets of light, have been referred to as 'Ch'i' or 'Qi' by the Chinese. Acupuncturists balance 'life force' or the yin and the yang. Jewish theosophy refers to the energy as Astral lights. Christian paintings often portray Jesus and other religious figures surrounded by a light energy. Native Americans and other cultures around the world have reported observing these energy fields. Count Wilhelm Von Reichenbach called it the 'odic' force. Wilhelm Reich named it the 'orgone.' Under a cloak of secrecy, the Russians conducted a considerable amount of research on the subject of subtle energies. Many of their findings are just now being released to the scientific community. In a future issue I hope to go into more detail concerning their work. For purposes of this report, suffice it to say that they have clearly demonstrated that the human body releases energy from its 'biofield' at frequencies between 300 and 2,000 nanometers.

"What makes this energy even more interesting, is the fact that it conforms to two laws of physics: sympathetic resonance and harmonic inductance. If this sounds too technical, bear with me. It's really not. You've probably seen these laws of physics demonstrated with tuning forks. After you strike a tuning fork, other tuning forks in close proximity will begin to vibrate at the same frequency and give off the same sound. In much the same way, diseased tissue or unbalanced groups of cells in your body can be brought back into harmony when exposed to the proper wavelength of energy.

"The MicroLight 830 laser unit emits photons at a frequency of 830 nanometers, which is apparently an effective wavelength for balancing the abnormal energy patterns associated with several conditions. These photons have been shown to activate enzymes, but only in cells in need of help (apparently those sending out energy at abnormal wavelengths). An enzyme, as you probably recall from high school chemistry, is a special molecule that remains totally intact, yet has the ability to speed up chemical reactions between other substances. Once an enzyme is activated, it starts a chain reaction of events. In the case of LLLT, the activated enzymes promote the repair and healing of damaged tissue in the area. The researchers involved in the General Motors study demonstrated that in addition to initiating the healing process, LLLT therapy also increased blood flow to the areas involved. (They thought even greater changes would be noticeable if there were a better method of monitoring blood flow at the microvascular and cellular levels.)

"LLLT is undoubtedly only one of many techniques that can be used to stimulate healing by balancing cellular energy. I suspect in the future we'll discover that certain types of music, homeopathy, acupuncture, massage, color therapy and a long list of other therapies work in much the same way. (Most of the therapies now used here at the Healing Research Center are used to create the same or similar effect.) For now, however, LLLT is on the forefront of modern, noninvasive therapy. It truly is the beginning of Star Trek medicine. The user doesn't have to have special abilities, talents or extensive training. It's safe. And most importantly, consistent results can be achieved by anyone using the proper equipment.

Star Trek Generation Doctors

"In my initial article on LLLT, I predicted that everyone would someday have one of these units in their home. Instead of running to the medicine cabinet for aspirin at the first sign of a headache or pain, the laser will be the first choice of treatment. After using the unit for close to two years now, I'll stick with that prediction. It seems like every day we're getting a little closer to realizing that subtle energies, like those emitted from these laser units, can have a profound effect on stimulating healing within the body. It's only a matter of time before physicians and the general public learn about LLLT and just how beneficial it can be.

"Low Reactive-Level Laser Therapy (LLLT) is alive and well. And while it is still far too expensive for the average consumer to own a unit, after using it for the last couple of years, I can't imagine a doctor's office without one. It's a therapy whose time has come. If you suffer from carpal tunnel syndrome, TMJ disorders, damaged nerves or any of the other conditions I've mentioned above, I would highly recommend seeking out a doctor who uses LLLT. In the large majority of these cases, it could very well eliminate the problem without the use of drugs or surgery."

Our Present Use of the Microlight 830

In our experience, we have had very few patients who have not received benefit from the MicroLight 830 and many have received truly outstanding help for conditions that had previously defied all other therapies.

The instructions that come with the device include protocols for the following: healing of open wounds; dermatitis; eczema; lack of granulation tissue formation (thus retarding wound healing); overcoming and softening scar tissue formation; fistulas; edema; cysts; bursitis; muscle inflammation, contusions, ruptures, atrophy and contractures; neuritis; neuralgia; nerve injuries; atrophy of nerves; paresis; paralysis;

prolapsed disc disease; spondylitis; periostis; spondylosis; bone fractures and fissures; arthritis, both rheumatoid and osteoarthritis; arthrosis; strains and sprains; dislocations (following reduction); tendonitis; epicondylitis; tendon strains and contusions; tendon ruptures and following tendon surgery; hematoma; tissue infiltration of blood after blood taking or injection.

Since the MicroLight 830 is stated to penetrate the tissues up to 30 mm (a little over one inch), we have used it over various ailing organs that we felt we could reach by this penetration. These include the liver, celiac nerve plexus (solar plexus), urinary bladder, inguinal hernia and prostate. Preliminary results of these efforts are very promising.

In the future we expect to find many new and fascinating uses for this little wonder. If you have a problem not very well served by previous treatments, feel free to ask your Healing Research Center physician about the MicroLight 830. It might well be the answer you have been searching for.

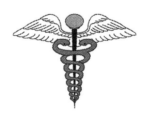

Index

misdiagnosis, 114
mold, 199, 258
mood changes, 281-282
mother–daughter (hereditary pattern), 6, 58-59
mother's milk, 22-23
immunization properties, 23
mouth, 33
mucus, 33
multiple sclerosis, 199
mumps, 179
muscle(s), 18-19, 26, 91, 93-94, 96, 141, 144-145, 205
involuntary contractions, 205
mass, 96
tension, 141, 144
tone, 18, 26, 94
weakness, 91, 93
Mycostatin, 188
myocardial weakness, 218-221
Myoflex, 123, 141-142, 164
myrrh, 191
myxedema, 18

N
natural products, 168
Nature Cure 2000, 165, 181
naturopathic care, xvi, 272, 279
nausea, 9, 14
neck, 143-144
neurasthenia, 16, 26-28
nerve-muscle-bone displacements, 143
nerve-muscle spasms, 143
nerve roots, 141
nervous system, 26-28, 43, 59-62, 74-76
neuroglandular mechanism/system, 1, 9, 11-12, 14, 26-27, 39, 59, 74-77, 108, 152, 214, 224-227, 281
exhaustion, 26-27
integrity, 59
sexual stability, 224-225
strength, 59
tone, 152
weakness, 26-27, 74-77
neurohormonal system, 1, 9, 11, 40, 44, 60, 70-72, 75, 92-98, 109, 126, 215, 227, 230

neurosis, 53
niacin, 165
nickel, 207, 212, 221, 269-270
toxicity, 207, 212, 269-270
occupational exposure, 269-270
signs and symptoms, 270
sources, 269
contact for allergic individuals, 269
nicotine, 203
nightshade family, 203
nitrogen excretion, 91, 96
Nizoral, 189
No-Doz, 203
"normal," 74-75, 108-109
nose, 33, 200-202
allergy, 200-201
lining, 200
membranes, 200-202
numbness of extremities, 27, 198
nutrition(al), 18, 49, 114, 123-127, 134, 161-175, 180, 284-285, 312
agents, 114
analysis, 163-169, 172-175
balance, 127, 164-169, 172, 174-175
compounds, 180
deficient(cies), 161, 168, 174-175
imbalance, diagnosing, 164
nutritional profile, 127, 167-169, 172-175
supplements, 123, 125-127, 161-175, 284-285, 312
minerals, 171-172
testing, 163-175
therapy, 125-127
nutritionist, 163-166
nuts, 246-247
Nystatin, 188-189

O
obsession, 57
old age, 16, 20-22
one cell–one antigen rule, of immune system, 242
One Flesh, 190, 223, 225, 227, 231, 234
"original sin," 225